The Theory and Practice of Group Therapy

Edited by Simon George Taukeni, Mukadder Mollaoğlu and Songül Mollaoğlu

Published in London, United Kingdom

The Theory and Practice of Group Therapy
http://dx.doi.org/10.5772/intechopen.106306
Edited by Simon George Taukeni, Mukadder Mollaoğlu and Songül Mollaoğlu

Contributors
Tirtha Prasad Mukhopadhyay, Armando Perez, Irina Katz-Mazilu, Mariangela Lippolis, Francesco Carlomagno, Fulvia Francesca Campo, Elvira Brattico, Esther Lynch, Jeremy Lynch, Kiela Hinson, Kayla Womack, Kiana McClintick, Bradford Pippen, Arturo Ezquerro, María Cañete, Mei-Ling Lin, Sherry H. Stewart, Emma E. Truffyn, Colin B. Pridy, Margo C. Watt, Amanda Hill, Mukadder Mollaoğlu, Songül Mollaoğlu

First published in London, United Kingdom, 2024 by IntechOpen
IntechOpen is the global imprint of INTECHOPEN LIMITED, registered in England and Wales, registration number: 11086078, 5 Princes Gate Court, London, SW7 2QJ, United Kingdom

British Library Cataloguing-in-Publication Data
A catalogue record for this book is available from the British Library

Additional hard and PDF copies can be obtained from orders@intechopen.com

The Theory and Practice of Group Therapy
Edited by Simon George Taukeni, Mukadder Mollaoğlu and Songül Mollaoğlu
p. cm.
Print ISBN 978-1-80355-675-8
Online ISBN 978-1-80355-676-5
eBook (PDF) ISBN 978-1-80355-677-2

For EU product safety concerns:
IN TECH d.o.o., Prolaz Marije Krucifikse Kozulić 3, 51000 Rijeka, Croatia,
info@intechopen.com or visit our website at intechopen.com.

Meet the editors

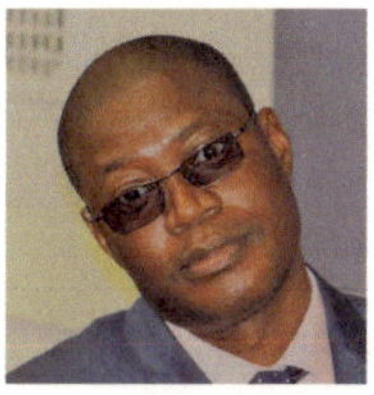

Simon George Taukeni is a professor, author, and editor working at the University of Namibia. He is a former post-doctoral research fellow at the University of Fort Hare, South Africa. Prof. Taukeni holds a Ph.D., MPH, MEd, a specialized post-graduate diploma in Behavioral and Emotional Disorder, and a BEd. He is the author of his autobiography *Against All Odds* and several edited books. Prof. Taukeni has also published numerous articles on diverse topics in health psychology, including psychosocial support, mental health, single-student mothers' dual roles, bereavement support, posttraumatic stress disorder (PTSD) among children, and more. He has collaborated with many local and international researchers and scholars as an editor, internal and external examiner, and principal project investigator. Prof. Taukeni is one of the pioneering scientists of the biopsychosocial model of health and he is a global citizen of note due to his impactful scientific contribution in Namibia, South Africa, and across the world.

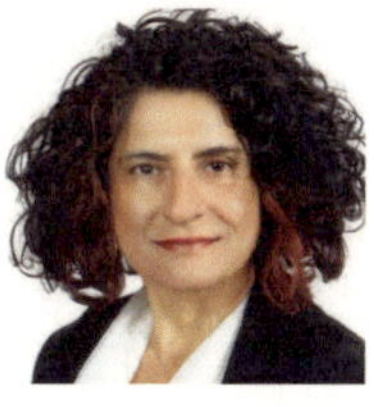

Professor Dr. Mukadder Mollaoğlu is a faculty member at the Faculty of Health Sciences, Sivas Cumhuriyet University, Turkey. Her research interests include care management in chronic diseases, quality of life, life satisfaction, home care, caregivers' needs, development of self-care activities in chronic diseases, integrative therapy, self-sufficiency, and health ethics. Her research work has been published in many high-impact journals and received numerous citations. She is an academic editor of book chapters and books. Professor Mollaoğlu received two first prizes, one in Sweden (Malmö) and the other in France (Strasbourg), for her work on life satisfaction and home care in chronic diseases. She also received the Lütfi Abay Culture and Education Foundation (LAKEV) science award in 2020 for her research in the field of health sciences.

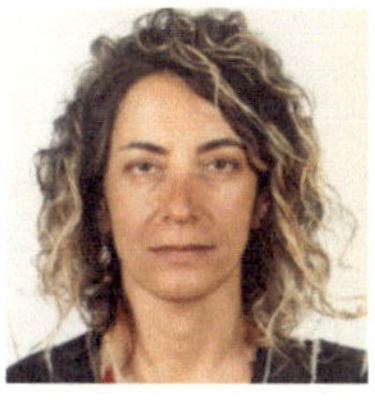

Dr. Songül Mollaoğlu graduated from Sivas Cumhuriyet University (SCU), Turkey, Education Faculty Fine Arts Department in 2005, and completed her master's degree in fine arts education at the Educational Sciences Institute of the same university in 2016. She completed her Ph.D. in Fine Art Education Program at Ankara University Institute of Educational Sciences in 2021 receiving the title of Associate Professor in 2022. She has authored many articles and book chapters on art therapy and semiotics.

Contents

Preface

Sometimes, individual effort may be required to cope with life's challenges and maintain inner balance. At this point, group therapy can offer people a different perspective. Group therapy, a type of psychotherapy that aims to help people manage mental health conditions or cope with negative experiences and behaviors, has a long history. Sometimes a group is established under a theme (weight loss, social phobia, addiction, etc.), while sometimes group treatment can be helpful for personal development. In this environment, group participants express their experiences and emotions, visualize their goals, and carry out planning activities to achieve them.

In music therapy, which can be applied individually or in groups, a music therapist works with a client or group in a planned manner to meet their physical, emotional, mental, social, and cognitive needs to achieve and facilitate communication, dialogue, learning, mobilization, expression, organization, and other related therapeutic goals. In a process, music and/or musical elements such as sound, rhythm, melody, and harmony are used. Therapeutic interventions aim to treat participants as a result of the neurophysiological effects of music on the organism. During the therapy process, music acts as a facilitator and, in some cases, a direct producer of the conscious and/or unconscious reactions and verbal responses of the participants in therapy.

This book is for professionals working in the health, social, and artistic fields, as well as therapists working in clinical settings.

We would like to thank all the authors who contributed to this book and the staff at IntechOpen, who provided invaluable cooperation and support throughout the publication process.

Simon George Taukeni
University of Namibia,
Windhoek, Khomas Region, Namibia

Mukadder Mollaoğlu
Faculty of Health Sciences,
Sivas Cumhuriyet University,
Sivas, Turkey

Songül Mollaoğlu
Faculty of Education,
Department of Fine Arts,
Sivas Cumhuriyet University,
Sivas, Turkey

Section 1

Group Therapy

Chapter 1

Perspective Chapter: Therapeutic Alliance, Rupture and Repair in Group Therapy

Esther Lynch, Jeremy Lynch, Kiana McClintick, Bradford Pippen, Kayla Womack and Kiela Hinson

Abstract

This chapter contains an overview of the therapeutic alliance including the purpose and importance of therapeutic alliance as well as recent research that provides knowledge on therapeutic alliance within the group therapy context. This chapter will also take a deep dive into understanding the rupture-repair model, its' connections with therapeutic alliance, and provide clinical examples of what a rupture and repair may look like in group therapy. Finally, this chapter discusses cultural considerations and includes clinical examples on rupture and repairs where individual and cultural differences are important. In conclusion, therapeutic alliance has been identified as a key contributor to positive outcomes for group therapy clients. While ruptures are expected to occur during therapy, It is important to note that both the rupture and the repair equally effect the therapeutic alliance as well as the outcome of treatment. Outcomes to therapy that align with a strong therapeutic alliance include reduced symptoms, client retention, improved outlook on life, and an improved occupational and interpersonal functioning. Outcomes of therapy associated with a successful repair involve a decrease in anxiety and depressive symptoms, increase in daily living activities, an increase in empathy for their group members, and stronger therapeutic alliance among the group.

Keywords: therapeutic alliance, repair, rupture, group therapy, cultural competence

1. Introduction

Many professionals consider therapeutic alliance to be a key hallmark of successful therapy. The quality of the working relationship or therapeutic alliance between the therapist and client is most beneficial when a strong bond is present, and the goals and tasks of therapy align. The core of exploring and understanding the therapeutic alliance is examining the client's attitude towards the therapist and the therapist's ability to engage and relate to the client. The two must mutually agree and collaborate on the goals and tasks of therapy, which takes understanding on both parts. Cultural competence plays an important role in the understanding process. Information must constantly be reviewed and evaluated for accuracy due to differences as well as similarities and how those experiences may or may not affect understanding.

This chapter explores the dynamics of therapeutic alliance in a therapeutic group setting. In a group setting the relationship or alliance exists within the whole group and the therapist leads the group through the therapeutic process.

In a group setting, there are many personalities to manage and to attempt to bring cohesion to the environment. When there is a breakdown in the alliance process, this is known as a rupture. Ruptures are a part of the process for both individual and group therapies. In a successful therapeutic alliance, the therapist and client, or group members can successfully resolve any tension or breakdowns in communication And successfully navigate difficulties in the collaboration of goals and tasks. If the rupture is not repaired correctly then it can lead to poor outcomes in therapy. We explore the types of ruptures that can occur as well as strategies to repair those ruptures correctly. Clinical examples are used to illustrate interventions used to manage ruptures and repairs to create a strong therapeutic alliance with group members.

2. Therapeutic alliance

There is a breadth of research about the benefits of alliance within therapy [1, 2]; Therapeutic alliance refers to the connection a therapist has with their clients and encapsulates a degree of trust and collaboration that sets the stage for future sessions [3]. More specifically, therapeutic alliance refers to the genuinely developed connection between therapist and client, and the degree of agreement and commitment to treatment goals used in treatment [4, 5]. A strong alliance exists when there is a strong foundational relationship that identifies each person's role in the relationship, and both agree on the goals and tools to be used.

Therapeutic alliance has emerged as one of the central contributors to positive outcomes for clients in therapy [3, 6]. The term therapeutic alliance was first mentioned by noted psychoanalyst Sigmund Freud and has since come to reflect Bordin's model, which emphasizes the need for clarity and collaboration [5]. A strong therapeutic relationship reflects the degree of agreement to working towards the mutually agreed upon treatment goals and clarifies the roles and expectations for both client and therapist [7].

Mental health professionals establish alliances with clients by providing space for vulnerability, conveying empathy, and remaining adaptable [8, 9]. Developing good therapeutic relationships requires working with the client to determine their goals while providing a judgment-free space. Additionally, studies have shown that a strong therapeutic alliance includes mutual agreement on the goals and tasks, and a willingness to make changes for the client's benefit [5, 8, 9].

2.1 Working towards alliance

Psychotherapists build strong therapeutic or working alliances with clients by establishing a sense of mutual respect, trust, and safety through social interactions [10]. Establishing and maintaining this connection requires the therapist to engage in an authentic working relationship geared towards helping the client reach specific, pre-identified goals for psychotherapy [11]. A strong therapeutic alliance exists between therapist and client when the client can express vulnerability openly [11].

The following example interaction illustrates how Joe, the therapist leading a group with the goal of developing effective communication builds alliance with the group by discussing individual goals during the first session [5].

Joe: Hello everyone and welcome to our first group session on developing effective communication skills. I'd like to start with everyone introducing themselves and giving a brief description of why you are here and what is your goal for becoming a part of this group.

Chris: Hello, my name is Chris and I'm here to improve my communication skills with the goal of communicating more effectively with my wife.

Kathy: Hi everyone. My name is Kathy and I decided to join the group so I could work to communicate more efficiently in my workplace.

Alice: Hi! My name is Alice, and I am here to work on my communication skills with the goal of repairing and improving my relationship with my adult daughter.

Although this interaction seems inconsequential, Joe knows how important it is and the impact it can make on therapeutic outcomes to develop therapeutic alliance with each individual in the group. Agreeing on the goals of treatment is one of the three essential elements that make up the therapeutic alliance [5].

2.1.1 Therapeutic alliance interventions

Interventions for establishing and maintaining therapeutic alliance in group psychotherapy include creating gender-specific groups, encouraging the formation of working relationships among members, treatment type, providing treatment options, words of encouragement from the psychotherapist-leader, and introducing mindfulness-based interventions [12–14].

In a systematic review of articles addressing therapeutic alliance, group cohesion, empathy, and goal consensus/collaboration in psychotherapeutic interventions, researchers found significant independent relationships between cohesion and rapport with positive treatment outcomes [13]. They also found studies that reported slightly increased collaboration was related to successful outcomes [13, 15]. However, a review of studies about collaboration in group psychotherapy found that this element may have an impact on treatment outcomes distinct from therapeutic alliance. The most notable impact on treatment outcomes were for those who were identified as being at risk for the likelihood of negative outcomes early on in treatment. The formal feedback during the collaboration helped to change the client's perception of change, motivation for treatment, the therapeutic relationship, and increase social support system [16].

2.2 Factors that affect therapeutic alliance

The climate of the relationship may have more impact on alliance building in group therapy than individual therapy [1, 14]. A meta-analysis of studies examining therapeutic alliance in group therapy and outcomes found a strong correlation specifically between the group leader-therapist and group members [1]. In other words, they found that the therapist's alliance with each group member was connected to their positive treatment outcomes [1]. However, when comparing the effects of alliance in group therapy compared to alliance in an individual therapy setting, results showed a slightly weaker for outcomes in group therapy. Though group therapy was found to have a slightly weaker effect on outcome than individual therapy, difference in the effect could be explained by the complex relationships that exist in group settings [1].

Another study found that individuals in group therapy pay more attention to the overall quality of their relationships with others in the group rather than everyone's assigned roles as member or leader [17]. Additionally, researchers found that the other versus self-focus factor present within group psychotherapy also influences therapeutic alliance building [18]. Meaning, the more members are interacting and focusing on the presenting concerns of their fellow group member, the stronger the group alliance will become.

The therapeutic alliance between group leaders, or psychotherapists, and group members, or clients, was found to be related to treatment outcomes in a Swedish study by Von Greiff and Skogens [19]. They examined positive changes in clients attending a group therapy program for alcohol and substance use. Clients' responses about acceptance, trust, confidence, and partnership revealed two themes identified as: 'treatment staff' and 'treatment group' [19, 20]. These themes align with the principles and goals of therapeutic alliance where the leader and its group members have an influence on treatment outcomes. A follow-up study by Von Greiff and Skogens [20] exploring the individual differences underlying clients' descriptions of alliance in a substance use psychotherapy group found that the social roles of clients impacted the group's cohesion. This study also found that race/ethnicity, social class, and particularly gender, can play a role in the psychotherapist-leader and client-group member relationship.

2.3 Treatment outcomes

Numerous studies have found a consistent link between therapeutic alliance and positive treatment outcomes for individuals in psychotherapy [21–23]. Specifically, the quality of the working alliance between therapist and client has been linked to successful treatment for a diverse array of clients, presenting problems, and treatment modalities [6, 21]. Four meta-analyses on therapeutic alliance conducted over two decades revealed a significant correlation between a strong working alliance between client and therapist and successful outcomes [21, 24, 25]. Although these studies examined alliances within the context of individual psychotherapy, a strong therapeutic relationship is similarly necessary for couples and group psychotherapy.

Successful outcomes connected to therapeutic alliance in psychotherapy include improved client retention, reduced symptoms, improved occupational and interpersonal functioning, and an improved outlook on life [22]. Researchers have examined the relationship between the working alliance of psychiatrists and patients and treatment outcomes [26]. Successful outcomes were evidenced by reported increased patient happiness with treatment, adherence to medication and keeping set appointments [22, 26]. Another study on therapeutic alliance between psychiatrists and patients with bipolar disorder resulted in fewer negative beliefs towards medication, diminished stigma towards bipolar disorder, and fewer manic symptoms [27]. These improved treatment outcomes are also connected to therapeutic alliance with psychotherapists.

Research focused on therapeutic alliance within group psychotherapy, or cohesion, has focused on various types of group relationships. One focus has been on the connection one member has with another member [1, 20, 28]. Findings show that individual relationships or working alliances between group members and the group leader play a significant role in group success [20, 28]. The relationship has more importance than the roles in the group.

2.4 Recent developments and future research

Though providing therapy online has existed for over 20 years, many mental health professionals first experience with teletherapy began during COVID-19.

Major reasons contributing to the resistance on doing therapy online include lack of experience, lack of training, unsuitable equipment, and difficulty managing ethical challenges. A recent study was conducted to understand the perception therapists had on building group therapy alliance online. Results showed that group therapeutic process, therapist comfort, and challenges predicted outcomes [29]. More specifically, the higher amount of therapeutic processes as well as therapist comfort level with online therapy, and the lower number of therapeutic challenges, the better the outcome. Another discovery was that group therapists reported lower satisfaction and comfort towards online therapy when comparted to in-person groups. Finally, this study reported that working through conflict and avoidance was more complicated for online groups. Even with complications, therapist continue to utilize technology to provide group therapy as even with these complications, it is evident the therapeutic processes found in face-to-face groups is also present in online groups.

Even with the breadth of research that exist on the topic of therapeutic alliance, large gaps in literature remain. Future research in this area could continue to the work of obtaining individual responses on clients and therapist to better understand how the alliance is being built, the nature of the alliance, and the overall outcomes of the therapeutic process in a qualitative nature. Future research could also lean towards a deeper investigation on the relationship between the therapeutic alliance and outcomes for specific diagnosis. Lastly, there is a lack of research focusing the culturally appropriate therapeutic alliance interventions.

3. Rupture and repair

Sometimes the communication and goals of the therapeutic approach are not aligned, and a rupture may occur in the therapeutic alliance. Any moments or period of times where breakdowns in the therapeutic alliance occur is considered to be a rupture. A rupture can be anything from a client disliking or disagreeing with something said, to a client not feeling that they are in a safe space where their deepest feelings and thoughts are free of judgment. A rupture can also include moments where a client withdraws when something is not said or addressed appropriately.

Ruptures and repairs are very common in sessions and can occur more than once during a session. Eubanks et al. [30] describes the process in which a rupture is repaired as a resolution process. This process allows the clients and therapist to work together to create therapy goals. The rupture should be addressed directly once it has been identified. Therapy cannot continue successfully if the therapeutic alliance is poor for long periods of time. The therapist may choose strategies like revealing their experience of the rift in the group or starting a new task [30]. Rupture resolution has been found to repair the harmful impact the experience may have brought on and repair the working alliance [31]. If a rupture and repair event is handled correctly, it helps to strengthen the relationship create a deeper bond. The rupture and repair event also gives insight into the client's interpersonal style, areas of defensiveness, and ability to handle conflict.

In a study conducted on clients with post-traumatic stress disorder, the researchers identified that ruptures in alliance were quite common (46%) [32]. As stated earlier, the therapeutic alliance can be a key factor in therapeutic outcomes for clients. As we understand what a rupture is in the context of a therapeutic relationship, we must also consider how our clients may feel if there is a rupture that is not repaired between the client and therapist [32], suggesting that the experience of an unrepaired rupture relates to poorer PTSD treatment outcome. Gersh et al., [33] identified a significant relationship between the time of the rupture in the therapy process. This study identified, in clients with borderline personality disorder, early treatment ruptures were associated with poor outcome whereas greater late treatment resolution was associated with better outcomes.

In this clinical example, Joe, Chris, Kathy, and Alice to show a rupture in a communication skills group setting evidenced by the client becoming defensive and rejecting the intervention [30].

Joe and Alice are discussing her fractured relationship with her adult daughter. Joe asks Alice if she was able to use the new communication skills they had discussed last week to attempt to resolve an argument she had with her daughter. Alice answers that she has not talked to her daughter this week. Joe asks, "Isn't one of your major goals for attending this group to repair your relationship with your daughter? Is there a reason why you chose not to reach out to your daughter this week?" Alice becomes visibly agitated and says, "I don't see how the new skill will help anyway. I'm not really sure why I'm here anymore. I don't appreciate you judging me, and I am not even the one who should be trying to repair the relationship. She is the one who ruined our relationship to begin with!"

3.1 Repair interventions

There have been a few interventions that therapists can use to repair alliance ruptures which center around the rupture and resolution model created by Safran and Muran [34]. Safran and Muran [34] stated that the interventions depend on metacommunication of the current situation. They referred to metacommunication as the act in which the therapist is constantly mindful of the client-therapist action. Safran and Muran [34] contributed to resolving therapeutic ruptures by creating direct and indirect interventions therapists can use. Direct interventions are considered as interventions where the client is actively engaged and aware of the intervention. Conversely, an indirect intervention are interventions that affect therapeutics alliance and covert in nature. Safran and Muran [34] suggested the following rupture resolution strategy model (see **Figure 1**).

A1a. Therapeutic Rationale and Tasks: This intervention consists of outlining or repeating the rationale of treatment [34]. If there is a rupture, therapists can check with clients to ensure they understand the goals and rationale of treatment and render explanations for clarity. Therapists can do this by employing therapeutic tasks/exercises that can help clients process therapeutic change.

A1b. Interpersonal Themes, Disagreements, and Tasks: Related to the goals and tasks of therapy, a client may disagree with the therapist, and it causes them to unintentionally process and explore interpersonal matters that may be affecting their treatment.

A2a. Clearing Misunderstandings: The therapist can clarify any misunderstanding a client may experience from therapy. This can look like the therapist helping the client resolve why they may feel a sense of discomfort.

A2b. Interpersonal Themes: Similar to A1b., this relates to how internal processes related to interpersonal matters can affect the bond between therapist and client.

B1a. Changing Goals and Tasks: The therapist works to change goals and tasks that are more relatable to the client(s) that that carry the possibility of increasing their willingness to participate in other tasks that more closely align with the therapist's goals for the group.

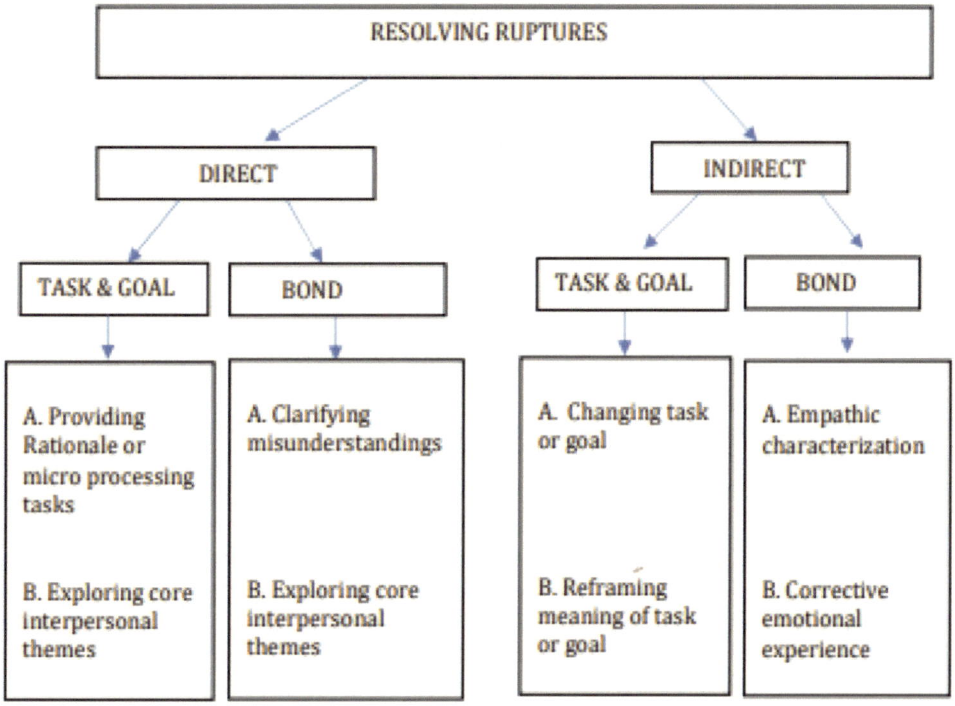

Figure 1.
Therapeutic alliance intervention strategies [32].

B1b. Reframing Goals and Tasks: This intervention involves reframing the goals and tasks to increase meaning and purpose for the client and increase the client's motivation to engage in the interventions.

B2a. Empathy: The therapist can take an empathetic approach and reframe the rupture in a positive outlook.

B2b. Emotional Experiences: The therapist can implicitly address the connection element of an alliance in a way that offers a different, beneficial interpersonal experience for the client.

Their goal in creating these strategies were to clear any misunderstandings among the group members and therapist, to adjust any goals and tasks of the group if deemed necessary, and to justify an intervention.

3.2 Treatment outcomes

Effective rupture resolution can impact the group, and other positive outcomes can be found [35]. Such positive outcomes include lessened anxiety and depressive symptoms, increase in daily living activities, and can lead to a stronger therapeutic alliance among the group. The group is provided with the tools necessary to move forward in the therapeutic process by sympathizing with other clients' issues and can lead the individual to see their negative self-appraisal of their internal beliefs [36].

In this repair example, Joe links Alice's defensiveness to the larger interpersonal communication patterns that have caused her problems in her past relationships [30] and works with Alice so she can recognize these patterns and develop alternative communication.

Joe takes a moment and nods. Joe says, "I assure you that my intention was not to judge you. I am curious, though, do you think that becoming defensive in the past has impacted your relationship with your daughter in a negative way?" Alice thinks about this carefully and says, "our last argument ended with me feeling judged and getting defensive with my daughter." Joe nods again and asks, "why do you feel the need to defend yourself in these situations? Are there other ways you can communicate what you need from the conversation without becoming defensive?"

3.3 Recent development and future research

Although there have been developments in psychotherapy research and practice with individuals, research in alliance ruptures and repairs regarding group psychotherapy is behind [35]. The challenge of research in groups is that the group structure is more complex than individual therapy. Group therapy offers a complicated set of interactions between members of the group, members to members, and group member to the therapist unlike individual therapy [36]. Unique to group therapy, interpersonal relationships and how they learn from one another is a factor to consider [18, 37]. It has been suggested that group psychotherapists can create a safe therapeutic environment by encouraging members who have experienced ruptures due to their interpersonal disregards (bitterness, intrusiveness, etc.) to bring the issue to the group, reflect on the ruptures impact on themselves and the rest of the group, and to learn positive ways to interact with the group members and therapist [18, 37]. A limited number of studies have investigated alliance in group therapy and no studies have explored the rupture and repair processes in real-time but instead have focused on alliance ratings within the group [35]. One current study by Garceau et al. [38], evaluated the usefulness and practicability of the Rupture Resolution Rating System (3RS) within a group psychotherapy context. This scale was used to explore whether and how the 3RS could apply to group therapy with a specific goal of assessing the interactions that occur in group therapy. Other goals included helping group therapists to better identify and repair rupture, informing research on the usefulness of managing ruptures and repair as they happen. Lastly, this study sought to identify possible modifications needed to make the 3RS compatible for the use of group therapy [38].

The 3RS is an observer-rated instrument system that is used to code ruptures and repairs in the individual psychotherapy context through videos or transcripts. The 3RS system counts the frequency in which there are withdrawal ruptures or confrontation ruptures. Withdrawal ruptures can look like the client "shutting down" or disengaging. Confrontation ruptures can look like the client challenging or controlling the therapist, or by confronting their frustrations. Once the codes are counted and rated, the session is then given an overall rating regarding the ruptures impact, how the ruptures were repaired, and the impact the therapist made on the ruptures [30, 39]. The instrument does not code every disagreement between the therapist and client as a rupture if the therapist and client acknowledge and discuss the rupture together [38]. As of this study, no other research has been conducted on the efficacy of using the 3RS system in a group psychotherapy setting.

4. Cultural considerations

To enhance group alliance, members and the group leader need to understand one another. Cultural differences play a role in the dynamics of understanding and building mutually agreed upon goals and tasks. Cultural competence was a term first introduced in 1989 by Dr. Terry Cross titled A Monograph on Effective Services for Minority Children Who Are Severely Emotionally Disturbed [40]. This piece of literature influenced the next generation of studies that investigated the impact of culture in systems of care. Since Cross [40], the integration of cultural competence into theoretical orientations, interventions, research approaches and methodologies has been expanded to more accurately address the impact of culture on outcomes [41–45].

The multicultural movement has been explained as the fourth major force in psychology behind psychoanalysis, behaviorism, and humanism [46]. The multicultural movement was developed in response to research that demonstrated mental health disparities among racial and ethnic minority groups [47]. In recent years, the exploration and investigation from the multicultural movement has required additional development and growth from clinicians. This growth requires a shift in the language of cultural competence into what is now understood as the framework of multicultural orientation [48]. The multicultural orientation framework centers three core concepts: Cultural Humility, Cultural Comfort and Cultural opportunities. Cultural humility includes recognizing that power differences exist between therapist and client on multiple levels, recognizing that these power differences include the power to define what is important and salient for others. The cultural humility framework also emphasizes the importance of understanding cultural differences influence assessment, diagnosis, treatment, and research [49].

Cultural comfort and cultural opportunities, the second and third core concept, are considered to be the behavioral representation of cultural humility. Cultural opportunities are indicators during therapy that provide an opportunity for the client's cultural identity to be explored [48]. These moments are usually initiated by the client and can involve their values and beliefs. Only when appropriate the therapist can also initiates a cultural explorative conversation. It is these conversations that lean into the concept of cultural comfort. Cultural comfort is defined as the mental and emotional experience therapist experience before, during, and after engaging in a cultural opportunity with their client. More specifically, cultural comfort is regarded as feeling open, calm, and present while also noting and accepting discomfort during culturally sensitive exchanges [48].

Hal et al., 2016 in their review of meta-analysis on cultural adaptations of psychological interventions found that, "culturally adapted interventions would produce greater reductions in psychopathology than another intervention or no intervention was supported" [50]. Hal et al., demonstrates the relationship between adapting or shifting interventions improves client psychopathology [50]. For example, a client may curse, or use swear words while responding during a group therapy session. Cursing can be an expression of the client's culture, experience and cursing can be an expression of culture [51]. The cultural responsiveness and humility of the counselor can provide an open stance to allow the client to communicate in the way that feels most comfortable to them [48]. This openness to allow the client to communicate in their own voice provides opportunity for deeper connection and improves the therapeutic alliance [52, 53].

The following clinical example illustrates a rupture where individual and cultural difference were important to attend to in a group setting as evidenced by a group member withdrawing from the group and from the work of therapy [30]. *Joe is a Black male therapist and is the leader of the group. The group is focused on developing effective communication skills. The group members include Chris, Kathy, and Alice. Chris is a 42-year-old White male. He joined the group with the goal to communicate more effectively with his wife. Kathy is a 37-year-old Black female. She became a part of the group to learn to communicate more efficiently in her workplace. Alice is a 53-year-old White female. Alice joined this group with the goal of developing her communication skills to assist in improving her relationship with her adult daughter.*

In this session, Joe, Chris, and Kathy are engaged in a group discussion. Kathy brings up an interaction she had at the airport earlier in the week. She expresses frustration because a security guard put his hands in her hair with no warning when she was going through airport security. Kathy expresses that this practice is discriminatory, dehumanizing, and disrespectful. The group can see that Kathy is visibly frustrated by this interaction.

Chris asserts, "Airport security searches everyone. I don't see how this practice is evidence of discrimination. They are just trying to keep us safe while flying." Chris then changes the topic to discuss an experience that he encountered this week that he was wanting to discuss with the group. Joe does not address this change in topic nor how Kathy's concerns are dismissed in this interaction. Kathy visibly withdraws from interactions with the group as the group continues to discuss how they used different communication skills throughout the week. This goes on for the rest of the session and this rupture is not addressed by Joe. Thus, Kathy feels unheard and invalidated both by other group members and by Joe, the facilitator of the group.

4.1 Repair

Though the research on repair within black, indigenous, and people of color (BIPOC) is scarce, the existing research does confirm engaging in the repair resolution process is integral to the rupture process within BIPOC population. A study completed by Yeo and Torress-Harding, found that microaggressions have a significantly negative effect on the therapeutic alliance [54]. Yeo and Torress-Harding also found that when therapist recognized, acknowledged, and invited a discussion of a rupture, where the therapist committed a microaggression towards the client, the therapeutic relationship was positively impacted [54]. Additionally, the participants emphasized a need for therapist to be more flexible in their approach, empathetic, and to increase their cultural sensitivity as well as knowledge.

The communication skills group that we observed in our earlier clinical example is meeting for their next session. In this example, Joe works to repair the rupture by acknowledging his contribution to the rupture [30] and apologizing for his role in the rupture. Joe also uses appropriate self-disclosure to bring discriminatory and uncomfortable search practices to the forefront of the conversation. Chris follows suit and also apologizes for causing the rupture by invalidating Kathy's experience. *Kathy is still actively withdrawn from the group, giving short answers only when necessary. Joe notices this and addresses his observations to the group, letting Kathy know that he has noticed her withdrawing from the group. It is clear that Kathy is visibly hesitant to answer, but after some time she says, "I was discussing what happened at airport security last session and my experience was dismissed by Chris." Joe says, "I'm sorry that your experience was overlooked last session and I apologize for not helping to maintain focus on your encounter." Joe looks at the group and asks, "has anyone here experienced discriminatory or even uncomfortable practices during a security procedure at an airport or elsewhere?" Chris and Alice shake their heads. Joe discloses, "I get 'randomly' searched frequently when I fly. I've never had anyone touch my hair in security, though. These experiences are not the same, but my experience does help me to be more empathetic regarding your incident. It is important to acknowledge that the intersection of your identity as a Black female isn't one that is shared by anyone in this group, and it is important for us to remember that when we are discussing different experiences. Chris, do you have any thoughts on the matter?" Chris takes some time to consider and then apologizes for dismissing Kathy's experience. Chris says, "I'm sorry that I didn't stop to think about how that experience made you feel. I also brushed off your assertion that the practice is discriminatory. Like Joe, I have never had my hair searched at airport security or anywhere else. Unlike Joe, I have never been randomly searched at airport security either."*

A key role in the therapeutic relationship is modeling the behavior that helps our clients tune in to and grow from the rupture and repair model [55, 56]. The relationship we have with our clients is both a reflection of their interactions with the outer world and a model for the type of behavior we wish to see our clients represent during and after the therapeutic process. The rupture-repair process in therapy better equips our clients with the ability to learn how to react, structure and respond to ruptures in other areas of their life. As helping professionals, clinicians have a responsibility to continue to develop our ability to understand various presentations of symptoms, diagnosis, and interventions accurately and critically.

5. Conclusion

The focus of this chapter is on understanding the role therapeutic alliance plays in group therapy. When a breakdown in the therapeutic alliance occurs, it must be addressed appropriately. This process is known as rupture and repair. The following are key areas to take away from this chapter.

- Therapeutic alliance has emerged as one of the central contributors to positive outcomes for clients in therapy. Having a strong therapeutic relationship reflects the degree of agreement in working towards the mutually agreed upon treatment goals and clarifies the roles and expectations for both client and therapist.

- Successful outcomes connected to therapeutic alliance in psychotherapy include improved client retention, reduced symptoms, improved occupational and interpersonal functioning, an improved outlook on life, increased client happiness with treatment, adherence to medication, and keeping set appointments.

- Research about therapeutic alliance within group psychotherapy, or cohesion, has focused on various types of group relationships such as the connection one member has with another. This indicates that individual relationships or working alliances between group members and with the group leader play a significant role in group success.

- Interventions for establishing and maintaining therapeutic alliance in group psychotherapy include creating gender-specific groups, encouraging the formation of working relationships among members, treatment type, providing treatment options, words of encouragement from the psychotherapist-leader, and introducing mindfulness-based interventions.

- Individuals in group therapy pay more attention to the quality of their relationships with others in the group rather than everyone's assigned roles as member or leader.

- The other versus self-focus factor present within group psychotherapy also influences therapeutic alliance building.

- Withdrawal ruptures can look like the client "shutting down" or disengaging. Confrontation ruptures can look like the client challenging or controlling the therapist, or by confronting their frustrations.

- Rupture resolution has been found to repair the harmful impact the experience may have brought on and repair the working alliance.

- Effective rupture resolution can impact the group, and other positive outcomes can be found. Those positive outcomes can include lessened anxiety and depressive symptoms, an increase in daily living activities, stronger therapeutic alliance among the group, and sympathizing with other clients' issues can lead the individual to see their negative self-appraisal of their internal beliefs.

- The 3RS is an observer-rated instrument system that is used to code ruptures and repairs in the individual psychotherapy context through videos or transcripts. The 3RS system counts the frequency in which there are withdrawal ruptures or confrontation ruptures.

- Though the research on repair within black, indigenous, and people of color (BIPOC) population is scarce, the existing research does confirm that engaging in the repair resolution process is integral when a rupture occurs.

Conflict of interest

The authors declare no conflict of interest.

Notes/thanks/other declarations

Many thanks to our loved ones and mentors for bringing us to this point of our journey.

Author details

Esther Lynch[1]*, Jeremy Lynch[2], Kiana McClintick[1], Bradford Pippen[1], Kayla Womack[1] and Kiela Hinson[1]

1 Tennessee State University, Nashville, United States of America

2 Fisk University, Nashville, United States of America

*Address all correspondence to: emendez@tnstate.edu

References

[1] Alldredge CT, Burlingame GM, Yang C, Rosendahl J. Alliance in group therapy: A meta-analysis. Group Dynamics: Theory, Research, and Practice. 2021;**25**(1):13. DOI: 10.1037/gdn0000135

[2] Ryu J, Banthin DC, Gu X. Modeling therapeutic alliance in the age of telepsychiatry. Trends in Cognitive Sciences. 2021;**25**(1):5-8. DOI: 10.1016/j.tics.2020.10.001

[3] Norcross JC, Lambert MJ. Psychotherapy Relationships That Work II. Psychotherapy. 2011;**48**(1):4-8. DOI: 10.1037/a0022180

[4] Ardito RB, Rabellino D. Therapeutic alliance and outcome of psychotherapy: Historical excursus, measurements, and prospects for research. Frontiers in Psychology. 2011;**2**:270. DOI: 10.3389/fpsyg.2011.00270

[5] Bordin ES. The generalizability of the psychoanalytic concept of the working alliance. Psychotherapy: Theory, Research & Practice. 1979;**16**(3):252

[6] Stubbe DE. The therapeutic alliance: The fundamental element of psychotherapy. Focus. 2018;**16**(4):402-403. DOI: 10.11176/appi.focus.20180022

[7] McParlin Z, Cerritelli F, Friston KJ, Esteves JE. Therapeutic alliance as active inference: The role of therapeutic touch and synchrony. Frontiers in Psychology. 2022;**13**:329. DOI: 10.3389/fpsyg.2022.783694

[8] Cameron SK, Rodgers J, Dagnan D. The relationship between the therapeutic alliance and clinical outcomes in cognitive behaviour therapy for adults with depression: A meta-analytic review. Clinical Psychology & Psychotherapy. 2018;**25**(3):446-456. DOI: 10.1002/cpp.2180

[9] Cameron SK, Rodgers J, Dagnan D. The relationship between the therapeutic alliance and clinical outcomes in cognitive behaviour therapy for adults with depression: A meta-analytic review. Clinical Psychology & Psychotherapy. 2018;**25**(3):446-456. DOI: 10.1002/cpp.2180

[10] Burke A. Four lessons in building therapeutic relationships. Counseling Today. 2021.Retrieved from https://ct.counseling.org/2021/11/four-lessons-in-building

[11] Pashak TJ, Heron MR. Build rapport and collect data: A teaching resource on the clinical interviewing intake. Discover. Psychology. 2022;**2**(1):20. DOI: 10.1007/s44202-022-00019-5

[12] von Greiff N, Skogens L. Positive processes of change among male and female clients treated for alcohol and/or drug problems. Journal of Social Work. 2017;**17**(2):186-206. DOI: 10.1177/1468017316638576

[13] Schnur JB, Montgomery GH. A systematic review of therapeutic alliance, group cohesion, empathy, and goal consensus/collaboration in psychotherapeutic interventions in cancer: Uncommon factors? Clinical Psychology Review. 2010;**30**(2):238-247. DOI: 10.1016/j.cpr.2009.11.005

[14] Wesson N. Center for the Study of Group Psychotherapy. Individual vs. Group Psychotherapy: how is the therapeutic process different? [Internet] Available from: https://csgp.org/blog/

individual-vs-group-psychotherapy-how-is-the-therapeutic-process-different/ [Accessed: December 1, 2023]

[15] Horvath AO. The alliance. Psychotherapy: Theory, Research, Practice, Training. 2001;**38**(4):365. DOI: 10.1037/0033-3204.38.4.365

[16] Tryon GS, Winograd G. Goal consensus and collaboration. 10.1037/a0022061

[17] Johnson JE, Burlingame GM, Olsen JA, Davies DR, Gleave RL. Group climate, cohesion, alliance, and empathy in group psychotherapy: Multilevel structural equation models. Journal of Counseling Psychology. 2005;**52**(3):310. DOI: 10.1037/0022-0167.52.3.310

[18] Yalom ID, Leszcz M. The theory and practice of group psychotherapy. Basic books; 2020

[19] Skogens L, von Greiff N. Recovery capital in the process of change—Differences and similarities between groups of clients treated for alcohol or drug problems. European Journal of Social Work. 2014;**17**(1):58-73. DOI: 10.1080/13691457.2012.739559

[20] von Greiff N, Skogens L. Understanding the concept of the therapeutic alliance in group treatment for alcohol and drug problems. European Journal of Social Work. 2019;**22**(1):69-81

[21] Flückiger C, Del Re AC, Wampold BE, Symonds D, Horvath AO. How central is the alliance in psychotherapy? A multilevel longitudinal meta-analysis. Journal of Counseling Psychology. 2012;**59**(1):10. DOI: 10.1037/a0025749

[22] Stanhope V, Barrenger SL, Salzer MS, Marcus SC. Examining the relationship between choice, therapeutic alliance and outcomes in mental health services. Journal of Personalized Medicine. 2013;**3**(3):191-202. DOI: 10.3390/jpm3030191

[23] Horvath AO, Del Re AC, Flückiger C, Symonds D. Alliance in Individual Psychotherapy[w:] Psychotherapy Relationships That Work: Evidence-Based Responsiveness. Norcross JC: Oxford University; 2011. pp.25-69. DOI: 10.1037/a0022186

[24] Horvath AO, Bedi RP. The Alliance, [w:] Psychotherapy Relationships That Work: Therapist Contributions and Responsiveness to Patients. Norcross JC: Oxford University; 2002. DOI: 10.1093/acprof:oso/9780199737208.003.0002

[25] Horvath AO, Symonds BD. Relation between working alliance and outcome in psychotherapy: A meta-analysis. Journal of Counseling Psychology. 1991;**38**(2):139. DOI: 10.1037/0022-0167.38.2.139

[26] Cruz M, Pincus HA. Research on the influence that communication in psychiatric encounters has on treatment. Psychiatric Services. 2002;**53**(10):1253-1265. DOI: 10.1176/appi.ps.53.10.1253

[27] Strauss JL, Johnson SL. Role of treatment alliance in the clinical management of bipolar disorder: Stronger alliances prospectively predict fewer manic symptoms. Psychiatry Research. 2006;**145**(2-3):215-223. DOI: 10.1016/j.psychres.2006.01.007

[28] Bernard H, Burlingame G, Flores P, Greene L, Joyce A, Kobos JC, et al. Clinical practice guidelines for group psychotherapy. International Journal of Group Psychotherapy. 2008;**58**(4):455-542. DOI: 10.1521/ijgp.2008.58.4.455

[29] Lo Coco G, Gullo S, Albano G, Brugnera A, Flückiger C, Tasca GA.

The alliance-outcome association in group interventions: A multilevel meta-analysis. Journal of Consulting and Clinical Psychology. 2022;**90**(6):513. DOI: 10.1037/ccp0000735

[30] Eubanks CF, Muran JC, Safran JD. Rupture Resolution Rating System (3RS). New York: Mount Sinai-Beth Israel Medical Center; 2015

[31] Stevens CL, Muran JC, Safran JD, Gorman BS, Winston A. Levels and patterns of the therapeutic alliance in brief psychotherapy. American Journal of Psychotherapy. 2007;**61**(2):109-129

[32] McLaughlin AA, Keller SM, Feeny NC, Youngstrom EA, Zoellner LA. Patterns of therapeutic alliance: Rupture–repair episodes in prolonged exposure for posttraumatic stress disorder. Journal of Consulting and Clinical Psychology. 2014;**82**(1):112. DOI: 10.1037/a0034696

[33] Gersh E, Hulbert CA, McKechnie B, Ramadan R, Worotniuk T, Chanen AM. Alliance rupture and repair processes and therapeutic change in youth with borderline personality disorder. Psychology and Psychotherapy: Theory, Research and Practice. 2017;**90**(1):84-104. DOI: 10.1111/papt.12097

[34] Safran JD, Muran JC. Resolving therapeutic alliance ruptures: Diversity and integration. Journal of Clinical Psychology. 2000;**56**(2):233-243. DOI: 10.1002/(SICI)1097-4679(200002)56:2%3C233::AID-JCLP9%3E3.0.CO;2-3

[35] Coco GL, Tasca GA, Hewitt PL, Mikail SF, Kivlighan JD. Ruptures and repairs of group therapy alliance. An untold story in psychotherapy research. Research in Psychotherapy: Psychopathology, Process, and Outcome. 2019;**22**(1):58-70. DOI: 10.4081/ripppo.2019.352

[36] Binder JL, Strupp HH. "Negative process": A recurrently discovered and underestimated facet of therapeutic process and outcome in the individual psychotherapy of adults. Clinical Psychology: Science and Practice. 1997;**4**(2):121. DOI: 10.1111/j.1468-2850.1997.tb00105.x

[37] Burlingame GM, Strauss B, Joyce A. Change mechanisms and effectiveness of small group treatments. Bergin and Garfield's Handbook of Psychotherapy and Behavior Change. 2013;**6**:640-689

[38] Garceau C, Chyurlia L, Baldwin D, Boritz T, Hewitt PL, Kealy D, et al. Applying the rupture resolution rating system (3RS) to group therapy: An evidence-based case study. Group Dynamics: Theory, Research, and Practice. 2021;**25**(1):89. DOI: 10.1037/gdn0000137

[39] Eubanks CF, Muran JC, Safran JD. Repairing alliance ruptures. 2019. 10.1093/med-psych/9780190843953.003.0016

[40] Cross TL. Towards a Culturally Competent System of Care: A Monograph on Effective Services for Minority Children Who Are Severely Emotionally Disturbed. Washington, DC: CASSP Technical Assistance Center, Georgetown University Child Development Center; 1989. DOI: 10.1037/pst0000160

[41] Brown LS. Cultural competence: A new way of thinking about integration in therapy. Journal of Psychotherapy Integration. 2009;**19**(4):340. DOI: 10.1037/a0017967

[42] Comas-Díaz L. Multicultural care: A clinician's guide to cultural competence. American Psychological Association.

Washington, D.C.; 2012. DOI: 10.1037/13491-000

[43] Guindon MH, Sobhany MS. Toward cultural competency in diagnosis. International Journal for the Advancement of Counselling. 2001;**23**(4):269-282. DOI: 10.1023/A:1014443901294

[44] Hayes SC, Muto T, Masuda A. Seeking cultural competence from the ground up. Clinical Psychology: Science and Practice. 2011;**18**(3):232

[45] Sue S. In search of cultural competence in psychotherapy and counseling. American Psychologist. 1998;**53**(4):440. DOI: 10.1037/0003-066X.53.4.440

[46] Pedersen PB. The making of a culturally competent counselor. Online Readings in Psychology and Culture. 2002;**10**(3):1-3. DOI: 10.9707/2307-0919.1093

[47] Sue DW, Bingham RP, Porché-Burke L, Vasquez M. The diversification of psychology: A multicultural revolution. American Psychologist. 1999;**54**(12):1061. DOI: 10.1037/0003-066X.54.12.1061

[48] Davis DE, DeBlaere C, Owen J, Hook JN, Rivera DP, Choe E, et al. The multicultural orientation framework: A narrative review. Psychotherapy. 2018;**55**(1):89

[49] Sylvia M. APA dictionary of psychology. CHOICE: Current Reviews for Academic Libraries. 2015;**53**(2):224-225. Available from: https://link.gale.com/apps/doc/A431198164/AONE?u=tel_oweb&sid=googleScholar&xid=6caffd67

[50] Hall GC, Ibaraki AY, Huang ER, Marti CN, Stice E. A meta-analysis of cultural adaptations of psychological interventions. Behavior Therapy. 2016;**47**(6):993-1014. DOI: 10.1016/j.beth.2016.09.005

[51] Goddard C. "Swear words" and "curse words" in Australian (and American) English. At the crossroads of pragmatics, semantics and sociolinguistics. Intercultural Pragmatics. 2015;**12**(2):189-218. DOI: 10.1515/ip-2015-0010

[52] Delgadillo J, Branson A, Kellett S, Myles-Hooton P, Hardy GE, Shafran R. Therapist personality traits as predictors of psychological treatment outcomes. Psychotherapy Research. 2020;**30**(7):857-870. DOI: 10.1080/10503307.2020.1731927

[53] Giffin HJ. Client's experiences and perceptions of the therapist's use of swear words and the resulting impact on the therapeutic alliance in the context of the therapeutic relationship[thesis]. Northampton Massachusetts: Smith College; 2016

[54] Yeo E, Torres-Harding SR. Rupture resolution strategies and the impact of rupture on the working alliance after racial microaggressions in therapy. Psychotherapy. 2021;**58**(4):460. DOI: 10.1037/pst0000372

[55] Bandura A. Psychotherapy as a learning process. Psychological Bulletin. 1961;**58**(2):143. DOI: 10.1037/h0040672

[56] Safran JD, Greenberg LS, Rice LN. Integrating psychotherapy research and practice: Modeling the change process. Psychotherapy: Theory, Research, Practice Training. 1988;**25**(1):1. DOI: 10.1037/h0085305

Chapter 2

Genesis and Development of Group-Analytic Therapy in Great Britain: Bion, Bowlby, Foulkes, and the Relevance of Group Attachment

Arturo Ezquerro and María Cañete

Abstract

A succinct account of the genesis and development of the Tavistock and group-analytic models of group psychotherapy focuses on their creators, Bion and Foulkes, and on how their life circumstances and their interpersonal and group attachment histories shaped their thinking and perception of the group and its therapeutic potential. The methodology combines historical investigation and literature review with psychodynamic and group-analytic formulations; it also provides an attachment-based, critical analysis of both approaches, their similarities and differences, and their mutual influence. Likewise, the chapter investigates the evolution of the concept of group attachment, formulated by Bowlby in 1969, which has been largely overlooked in the specialist literature until the last two decades, despite the fact that group lives, as well as interpersonal and group attachment, have played a fundamental role in our survival as a species and in our well-being and healthy development as a person. The present research is also informed by anthropological, psychosocial, organisational, and cultural aspects of human growth. It concludes that group attachment is highly relevant to group psychotherapy and that studying its nature and therapeutic implications should be an integral part of the training of psychotherapists and other mental health professionals, particularly those working with groups.

Keywords: Bion, Bowlby, Foulkes, development, group analysis, group attachment, group psychotherapy, survival, Tavistock model

1. Introduction

Groups are at the core of human existence and survival; for millions of years, they have been fundamental for healthy development and have contained healing properties. Today, optimally, we may define group psychotherapy as a democratic, cost-effective, and inclusive form of psychosocial treatment.

In fact, from the outset, group therapy has been strongly connected to survival, both physical and emotional. It is widely accepted that this treatment modality was pioneered by the American medical doctor Joseph Pratt in 1905, as he decided to put together a number of patients with pulmonary tuberculosis in Greater Boston: there was a life-threatening illness to fight.

These patients were segregated from the community, in a way similar to the many forms of discrimination and marginalisation inflicted upon patients suffering from serious mental illness.

Pratt actually thought that, for his patients, sharing the knowledge of their illness and their coping strategies would not only provide them with much-needed emotional support, but would also help them maximise their chances of survival.

Indeed, these group therapy sessions were complemented with a psychoeducational component, largely delivered by Pratt himself [1]. This combined approach raised an important issue about how to integrate harmoniously the *authority* of the leader with the *authority* of the group.

Interestingly, Pratt was not a psychiatrist or mental health professional, but an internist. Somehow, this speaks in favour of the universality and healing potential of group processes, as well as the fact that mind and body are inextricably linked.

Some of the techniques used at the time can still be found in a range of group therapeutic interventions today, particularly in homogeneous groups, in which all patients have a common condition.

In Great Britain, the birth of group psychotherapy had its own specific intensity and purpose, in the context of the Second World War. There was an overwhelming and urgent problem to solve: having to fight and survive the war. That was, undeniably, a group effort.

At a psychological and political level, and in different ways, the task of developing group therapy was greatly facilitated by the work and ideas of three leading figures: Wilfred Bion, SH Foulkes, and John Bowlby, as we will see throughout this chapter.

In 1952, the Group Analytic Society International (GASI) was created and, in 1971, the Institute of Group Analysis (IGA) started national training programmes, based in London.

From its inception, IGA (a member of the European Group-Analytic Training Network) has offered a comprehensive training in adult group psychotherapy. In order to qualify as an IGA group analyst, current requirements include a one-year introductory course, followed by a one-year diploma course and a three-year qualifying course.

Apart from the training requirements of attending academic seminars, writing clinical and theoretical dissertations, and receiving their own personal group therapy, trainees have to conduct on their own (under supervision) a heterogeneous and slow-open mixed group with adults who are strangers to each other. In addition, they must conduct a special interest group, which can be homogeneous and might involve children, adolescents, adults or older adults.

Malcolm Pines [2], a founding member of both GASI and IGA, suggested that, in therapy groups as well as in other group configurations, members (including the therapist, conductor, or leader) share a common space: the powerful universal symbol of the circle, which has been a setting for the development of human relatedness through our evolution as a species.

Certainly, we can imagine our distant ancestors sitting in a circle around a comforting fire, after a long day, sharing true stories and fantasies, forming a natural (therapeutic) group and growing in their group belonging or affiliation and, also, in their *group attachment*, a more than useful concept outlined by Bowlby [3], the *father* of attachment theory. We shall elaborate on this later.

DOI: http://dx.doi.org/10.5772/intechopen.111826

Mark Ettin [4], the inaugural recipient of the American Group Psychotherapy Foundation's award for excellence, also referred to the healing properties of the group circle, about which he described a number of poetic metaphors. He pointed out that, in some religious traditions, circular motion has symbolised the sweeping, spinning, and stirring process of creation.

Furthermore, in some primitive communities, dancing a round (along a circle) was thought to animate the still forces of nature. Roundness became a sacred shape and evolved into a universal symbol of wholeness, a major goal in human developmental processes across the life course [5].

Likewise, the circle was associated with other healing properties, such as its inherent potential for mixing, arranging, and enveloping disordered and polarised multiplicities. The early psychoanalyst Carl Jung [6] suggested that, in a circular configuration, pointed edges can be smooth, relationships circumscribed, splits conjoint and chaos contained.

Other authors [7, 8] likened the group to the good-enough environmental mother, and equated the group's reliable felt presence with an internally held comforting mother image: an archetype representing the holder of life.

In the following sections of this chapter, we will explore the genesis and development of the two main methods of group psychotherapy in Great Britain, which were pioneered by Bion and Foulkes. They created two distinct approaches, respectively: the Tavistock model and the group-analytic model.

Moreover, in this study, we shall describe and critically compare both approaches from our first-hand perspective, having trained in both institutions: the Tavistock Clinic and the IGA. In addition, we will explore Bowlby's group mind, as well as core tenets of his attachment theory (such as the concept of group attachment) and his contribution to the field of group therapy.

2. Historical context to group therapy in Britain. Part I: the Tavistock model

Prior to the Second World War, in the UK and in other European countries, group psychotherapy was viewed by many members of the mental health community with a variety of negative feelings, which ranged from doubt to suspicion to contemptuous rejection. The primacy of the one-to-one therapeutic relationship and the analysis of the so-called *transference neurosis* were seen as central elements in any form of psychodynamic psychotherapy [1].

After the war, the use of the group as a method of treatment flourished in its own right, despite early hostile attitudes. There were many reasons for this. For example, in the context of war calamity and its aftermath, the group approach made it possible for more people to be treated by the same number of therapists.

And group psychotherapy gradually came to be a highly cost-effective and beneficial form of treatment for many different conditions in a wide range of settings [5].

In 1946, Wilfred Bion (1897–1979) was put in charge of group psychotherapy at the Tavistock Clinic, in London. Like most of his colleagues over there, he qualified as a psychoanalyst in the post-war years and was strongly influenced by Melanie Klein.

Bion had a charismatic personality, despite having experienced a difficult interpersonal attachment and group attachment history. His parents (to whom he felt insecurely attached) sent him to England for his education as a young child, whilst they remained in India contributing to the might of the British Empire at its pick.

After the separation from his parents, he missed home, struggled at a very strict boarding English school, sustained a serious physical injury whilst playing rugby and, later, went through severely traumatising experiences during the First World War [5].

At the age of just under 18, Bion joined the British Royal Tank Regiment. He became a Brigade Major at 19 and was sent to France where he was on active service until the end of the war. It seems that his military experience and reputation played an important part in the development of his charismatic thinking, and in the perception that other people had of him during his later professional career.

In those early days, more often than not, tanks were death traps from which only few survived. The following episode, whilst Bion was in charge of a group of tanks, became legendary. The day before one of the battles, he objected to the order of an attack in daylight, because he considered it would be suicidal. He suggested to attack either at dawn or dusk, with the cover of some mist.

This occurred at a time when higher commands new little about the handling of tanks. Following Bion's objection, the divisional commander responded firmly, as reported by Trist [9]:

> *Wilfred, you may be one of my best officers but you are a boy. You may know more about these new machines than I do but you know less about battles. We will attack at 10 o'clock.*

Bion rose again and said:

> *Sir, as I am a soldier, I obey orders and will attack at 10 o'clock, but as a staff officer I have the right to have my technical advice recorded in writing in the minutes of this meeting. You neglect it at your peril.*

The following day, the tanks were wiped out; only Bion came back. In *The Long Week-End* [10], there is a moving autobiographical description of the fear and trauma of battle, looking back to that tragedy. He went further than that and actually wrote that his life concluded then.

We can imagine the deep sense of trauma Bion might have gone through, as he struggled to recover from the horror of the carnage of his companions, whilst he was also trying to make sense of his own survival. Interestingly, in his later professional life, he conceived a good therapist as one who has developed a capacity to think *under fire*. Surely, this conception relates both metaphorically and literally to the above war experiences.

It should be noted that the Tavistock Clinic opened in 1920, largely in connection with the need to provide psychological support to members of a society deeply traumatised by the First World War. However, at the time, the institution only offered individual psychotherapy.

Some 25 years later, when the Second World War had ended, there was an exponential increase of patient referrals. This pushed the Tavistock Clinic's management to develop therapeutic methods that would help the institution meet such an overwhelming demand.

With the arrival of the National Health Service (NHS) in 1948, the Clinic was under pressure to maintain a patient-load sufficiently large, as to satisfy the new NHS authorities that out-patient psychotherapy would be helpful and cost-effective [11].

In fact, by the time the Clinic entered the NHS, many of the senior staff were already running patients groups under Bion's headship. He also conducted groups for industrial managers and professionals from the educational world. In order to attract patients for the therapy groups, he offered two options: to wait 1 year for individual treatment or to start group treatment immediately [12].

In the early years, the strategy worked and there was strength in numbers. Bion was very enthusiastic about injecting his group ideas into the Tavistock's post-war culture. Neurosis started to be perceived as a problem of personal relationships and, therefore, it had to be treated as a group phenomenon rather than as a purely individual one [13, 14].

Some of the Clinic's new staff accepted that group psychotherapy was a most timely development, at a key moment when war survivors needed to learn how to help one another. Bion based his group therapy programme on his conception of man as a *political animal*, as he put it:

> *... an animal whose fulfilment can only approach completeness in a group. (Bion, in [11], p. 144)*

However, there were difficulties getting in the way. Henry Dicks further pointed out that the newly-elected Tavistock's professional committee knew pretty well what the views of most colleagues on the old staff were:

> *... disapproval of group therapy; there was difficulty in understanding that a community view of psychiatric disorders did not imply disrespect for the sanctity of the individual therapeutic relationship. ([11], p. 154)*

Despite being a hugely influential and captivating figure, Bion gradually started to lose control of the situation. Perhaps he employed too radical an approach, as he seemed to be treating only the group as-a-whole, as if it were a single individual, rather than treating the individual group members. Many patients deserted or dropped out of group treatment.

Bion, who presented himself as the *only* source of *authority* in his therapy groups, might have been disappointed with the therapeutic results or unhappy with the sceptical culture towards groups within the institution, or both.

In any case, by 1952, he gave up and stopped running groups for patients at the Clinic or elsewhere [9]. However, he delegated his leadership of the Tavistock's group therapy programme to Henry Ezriel and Jock Sutherland, who thoroughly described the application of Bion's ideas as a method of psychoanalytic group therapy.

Ezriel [15–17] and Sutherland [18] favoured a technique whereby nothing but rigorous group-as-a-whole, here-and-now transference interpretations need be used. Ezriel particularly considered that these interpretations had to be delivered in the same manner as in individual psychoanalytic sessions. In this approach, the group became a *quasi-individual*.

For several decades, the overall mood in the institution was that therapy groups did not work. In the mid-1970s, David Malan led a comprehensive piece of research: 42 randomly selected patients were interviewed 2–14 years after termination of psychoanalytic group therapy at the Tavistock Clinic. The findings were staggering [19]:

Comparison of psychodynamic changes in patients who stayed less than 6 months with those who stayed more than 2 years gave a null result. The majority of patients were highly dissatisfied with their group experiences. However, there was a strong positive correlation between favourable outcome and previous individual psychotherapy.

These results cast doubts on the appropriateness of transferring to group treatment the strictly individual psychoanalytic approach, and critically pointed at the stringent approach employed by Bion and his followers. By the late 1970s, there was a sharp decline (almost extinction) of group psychotherapy at the Tavistock Clinic.

However, with some modifications, the Tavistock model was beginning to pick up at the time we started our training at the Tavistock Clinic, in the mid-1980s.

This revival owes a great deal to the work of Sandy Bourne, who allowed for his group therapy sessions to be observed behind a one-way screen (followed by clinical discussions) as a learning method, and to Caroline Garland [20], who had recently completed her group-analytic training at the IGA (*next door*) and brought a newly found sense of enthusiasm and creativity to the Tavistock.

Both Bourne and Garland played a large part in the process of re-engaging the institution with a revised, more user-friendly, evidence-based, methodologically stronger, and more effective philosophy of psychoanalytic group therapy.

3. Historical context to group therapy in Britain. Part II: the group-analytic model

In contrast to the Bionian or Tavistock model, SH Foulkes (1898–1976), a German-born psychiatrist and psychoanalyst who came to England as a refugee, paid specific attention to the individual needs of his group patients, whilst keeping in mind the group as-a-whole and claiming that, ultimately, the individual is an *abstraction* and cannot exist outside a group.

Foulkes [21–24] developed the group-analytic approach, in which the therapist or conductor usually provides *security* and *immunity* for as long as the group is in need of them. Like Bion [10, 13, 25], he also conceived man as a social animal whose fulfilment can only achieve completeness in a group.

However, Foulkes's therapeutic attitude comprised more distinct holding and containing qualities, towards both the group itself and the different individuals within it. For this, he took into account other levels of group life, such as its intrinsic sociability, together with conscious and unconscious understandings that people in the group-analytic *matrix* demonstrate to each other. He believed in the *inner-authority* of his patients.

Whilst Bion was largely influenced by Melanie Klein, Foulkes's primary influence was Sigmund Freud [26], who himself had concluded that the psychology of the group is the oldest human psychology. This theoretical contrast between Bion and Foulkes was amplified by the differences in their real-life experiences.

Foulkes had a more benign interpersonal attachment and group attachment history than that of Bion. He was brought up in the prosperous city of Karlsruhe, in a liberal and middle-class Jewish family. He experienced sufficiently secure attachments with both his parents; he was a popular boy at school, and thoroughly enjoyed playing football and tennis [27].

At the age of 18, Foulkes was enlisted in the telephone and telegraph section of the German Army, during the First World War. He served in France in the rear, where he discovered the power of *communication* for maximising survival. This idea would become one of the cornerstones of his conception of group psychotherapy [28, 29].

After the war, Foulkes undertook his psychiatric training in Berlin and his psychoanalytic training in Vienna. But his career and his family life were disrupted by the Nazi danger. Together with Erna (his first wife) and their three children, he had to run away from Germany to the relative safety of the UK, in order to evade an order that Hitler dictated in 1933 for him to surrender his passport.

Upon his arrival in London, he changed his German-Jewish name (Siegmund Heinrich Fuchs) to a phonetically British one, in order to disguise his identity of origin and, thus, maximise his chances of survival. Officially, he became SH Foulkes. In addition, he asked his family and friends not to use his first or middle name, but to call him Michael [30].

With the outbreak of war, London was no longer a safe place and Foulkes moved to the provincial town of Exeter, where he led his first therapy group in 1940. This group was made up of a number of patients he was treating individually. He felt curious about what they may have to say to each other if they were put together as a group. Indeed, he was experimenting, as Pratt had done some three decades earlier. And he also did it with a *safety net*.

In the group, Foulkes [22] listened to the conversations of his patients with a technique that he would later describe as *free-floating attention*, a kind of equivalent to the *free association* of the individual psychoanalytic method.

He also paid attention and tried to be sensitive to how the words were expressed and connected to one another (or otherwise), including the tone and modulation of the voice and the non-verbal language. That was the birth of what is known today as group-analytic psychotherapy.

Generally speaking, Foulkes [23] conceived his therapeutic role as that of a conductor and facilitator of communication and understanding amongst group members. In fact, he emphasised that the most important factor in group therapy is the process of communication itself, rather than the mere information that is transmitted.

Over time, perhaps influenced by his work as a *communicator* during the First World War, his views became quite radical, suggesting that psychotherapy is about keeping the communication process alive. Therefore, in his mind, psychotherapy and communication came to be the very same thing.

There was another important background to the evolution of his ideas. In 1943, Foulkes was called up as a British Army medical officer to replace Wilfred Bion and John Rickman, who had jointly led a therapeutic project called the First Northfield Experiment. Northfield was a military psychiatric hospital near Birmingham, in the heart of England.

This hospital had been reorganised with a view to helping the Army identify which soldiers had the possibility of making a recovery from their mental problems, in order to return to the front lines, and who should be discharged as unrecoverable.

The usual diagnosis used at that time was *shell shock* or *war neurosis*; what is now called post-traumatic stress disorder had not yet been clearly conceptualised.

Bion and Rickman [14] had introduced a radical treatment regimen. Neurosis was seen as the enemy; soldiers had to learn to face such an enemy and develop the courage to pick up their rifles again.

It would appear that Bion and Rickman tried very hard to get sick soldiers back on active duty as quickly as possible, perhaps without fully addressing their mental health problems. Since the war context had generated highly dangerous and critical situations, from their point of view, the survival of the group and that of the nation had priority over the survival of the individual.

For reasons not entirely clear, this first group therapy project crashed before taking off. The military authorities, puzzled by the disturbance caused within the hospital environment, decided to close it down after only 6 weeks [5].

We have the impression that Bion and Rickman failed to anticipate the tremendous impact of their drastic measures, not only on the sick soldiers but also on the therapeutic community they were trying to create. However, they laid key theoretical foundations, which turned out to be seminal for the study of group dynamics, both in therapeutic and institutional contexts across the world [13, 25].

Soon after Bion and Rickman left, Foulkes set up a new programme, called the Second Northfield Experiment. He incorporated some of the notions of his predecessors, but used group psychotherapy more specifically for the emotional well-being of soldiers than as a tool for returning them to the battlefields to face death.

His attitude was so benign that he often began a group therapy session with the following remark:

> *As long as we are in this psychotherapy group, we are not in the Army. (Foulkes, cited in [27], p. 203)*

Although Northfield's two experiments differed in pace, technique, and effectiveness, they both shared many underlying concepts, such as social responsibility and the therapeutic use of the environment or milieu. In other words, both Bion and Foulkes perceived the hospital as-a-whole and tried to develop its healing potential as a therapeutic community [2].

Despite his doubts and hesitations, Foulkes made Northfield's second experiment a success. From 1943 to 1945, he treated vast numbers of soldiers, all in groups, as psychiatric casualties in the Army came to increase on a massive scale. With care and patience, Foulkes designed an innovative and powerful psychotherapeutic tool [27].

Although he drew heavily on psychoanalytic ideas, his technique was not a direct application of psychoanalysis to the group, but a form of therapy, *in* the group, and *by* the group, including its conductor [21–23].

This Foulkesian conception is similar to what has been called second-order cybernetics, in which the observer is part of what is observed or treated [30].

In this way, Foulkesian group-analysis gradually became an idiosyncratic therapeutic philosophy. In this philosophy, patients are conceived as possessors, not only of problems, but also of sufficient internal resources to help each other and, ultimately, become a *group of co-therapists* [31].

It is true that Foulkesian theory has often been criticised as vague or imprecise, even within group analysis itself. However, this vagueness or imprecision has been perceived by others as one of its strengths and a valuable element, since it avoids dogmatism and adapts relatively flexibly to the needs of the patient.

Over time, group analysis has become a solid theoretical and clinical discipline, particularly with regard to the study of interpersonal, intragroup, and intergroup relationships and their therapeutic potential (in small, medium and large groups), as well as to the promotion of healthier communities [5].

In recent decades, group analysis has extended its approach to the study of social thought, power dynamics and political tensions [32], as well as the so-called collective or social unconscious [33].

4. Bowlby's conception of group attachment

John Bowlby (1907–1990) was born in London only 6 years after the death of Queen Victoria. He was brought up in an upper-middle-class family where Victorian tradition was the norm. He could not establish secure attachment relationships with his parents, who left his care to a nursemaid with whom he developed an intimate attachment. However, he lost her before the age of four—a departure that he considered almost as tragic as the loss of a mother [12].

Bowlby was only seven when the First World War erupted. His father was immediately sent off to the Front. During the course of the war, Bowlby and his brother Tony were dispatched to boarding school because of the danger of air raids on London or, at least, that was what they were told. As an adult, he reflected that it was just an excuse, as part of a traditional step in the time-honoured barbarism required to produce English gentlemen [34].

Sometime later, Bowlby indicated that he had been sufficiently *hurt* but not sufficiently *damaged*, as a result of his childhood experiences. Although he never criticised his parents, his views on the attachment needs of young children could be seen as an indictment of the type of upbringing to which he had been subjected and of the culture that had fostered it [30].

In 1946, the very same year Wilfred Bion had set up the Tavistock Clinic's group therapy programme, and in competition with Donald Winnicott, John Bowly (who had trained as a child and adolescent psychiatrist and as a psychoanalyst) was appointed as Chair of the Children and Parents Department at the Clinic.

In the early days, Bowlby was significantly influenced by Bion, but he developed his own way of applying group methods therapeutically. In fact, he laid the foundations of therapeutic group work with families, by seeing all members of the family together. And he described his work in a ground-breaking paper, *The study and reduction of group tensions in the family* [35], the first European publication in the field of family therapy.

In addition, Bowlby established a weekly therapy group for mothers and their babies or young children, which he called the *Well-Baby Clinic*. He put aside one afternoon, every week, for this group therapy project and conducted it during the course of three decades.

Not unexpectedly, group membership changed when some mothers improved and were replaced by others. He succeeded in creating a therapeutic group dynamic and culture. And he gave priority to:

> *... trying to help the less experienced learn from those who knew more. ([36], p. 29)*

However, Bowlby [3, 37–41] became so involved in his research into the nature of the child's tie to his mother and, subsequently, into the evolutionary roots and functions of human attachment throughout the life cycle, that he did not provide a detailed account of his group-therapy clinical findings, nor did he link these to his attachment theory.

At one point, he confessed that he left to others the task of integrating group therapy and attachment-based thinking [5].

Another major contribution of John Bowlby was the creation of the first research unit at the Tavistock Clinic. He promoted an aspiration that a research component should be built in to all current and future therapeutic work. That was with the aim of refining knowledge and feeding the conceptual refinement back into the subsequent clinical activities of the institution: no research without therapy and no therapy without research [11].

According to Bowlby [3, 41], attachment (like food and sexuality) is a fundamental and integral part of our existence and survival, all the way from the cradle to the grave. The strength of the instinctual component of attachment gradually allows for the establishment of meaningful, intimate and enduring interpersonal and group attachment relationships.

John Bowlby was no doubt a group person who conceived the human mind as a social phenomenon. Whilst he originally investigated the nature of the child's attachment to the mother within the family environment [37–39], the compass of his work included other manifestations of interpersonal attachment and of group attachment through other developmental stages in the life cycle:

> *During adolescence and adult life, a measure of attachment behaviour is commonly directed not only towards persons outside the family but also towards groups and institutions other than the family. A school or college, a work group, a religious group or a political group can come to constitute for many people a subordinate attachment figure, and, for some people, a primary attachment figure. In such cases, it seems probable, the development of attachment to a group is mediated, at least initially, by attachment to a person holding a prominent position within that group. ([3], p. 207)*

Inevitably, humans are born into a group. From birth onward, infants start to internalise group experiences, either directly or through their interactions with their attachment figures, who have mental representations of their own previous group experiences. In our evolution as a species, the group became an adaptive social organisation in the service of survival. The group is a humanising environment *par excellence*, and can also be a therapeutic and attachment space [42].

Undeniably, attachment theory is firmly grounded on Darwin's theory of evolution. Primarily, attachment serves survival (both physical and emotional) and gradually becomes the basis for healthy psychosocial development throughout the life cycle. Attachment is both an in-built force for human connectedness and a significant relationship that makes life more meaningful:

> *Intimate attachments to other human beings are the hub around which a person's life revolves, not only when he is an infant or a toddler or a schoolchild but throughout his adolescence and his years of maturity as well, and on into old age. From these intimate attachments a person draws his strength and enjoyment of life and, through what he contributes, he gives strength and enjoyment to others. ([41], p. 442)*

5. Discussion

We have suggested elsewhere [5] that Bion's traumatic experiences during the two world wars and his difficult interpersonal and group attachment history contributed to his conception of the individual as a group animal who is at war with his *groupishness*—an assumption which he did not revise and which, in many ways, became deified and dogmatised.

Foulkes also had to endure trauma, but he was able to establish more secure interpersonal and group attachments. His group-analytic mentality, the *matrix*, is not at war with the individual. According to him, the broad range of negative and positive responses generated in a well-functioning group enhances, both, the person's individuality and groupality.

This *group matrix*, with its emphasis on a deepening of group members' capacity for personal insight and mutual understanding through their own contributions, as well as those of the conductor, adds a more democratic therapeutic dimension or group culture that is lacking in the defensive *group mentality* that Bion [25] had originally conceptualised.

In terms of attachment theory, the therapeutic *group matrix* (including members and the therapist or conductor) has been described as constituting a *secure base* or, at least, a secure-enough base [5, 12, 43–46].

In its purest form, Bion's technique provokes a significant amount of frustration; it may lead to disappointment, even hostility. However, this is not necessarily a bad thing; after all, learning to tolerate frustration without resorting to destructive anger and aggression is an important developmental task.

Having said that, too much frustration and disappointment can generate unbearable levels of anxiety and dysfunctional, even aggressive, group mentalities—particularly in the more vulnerable patients.

Foulkes gathered that, as well as repressed hostility, patients bring a feel for group connections, collaboration and meaningful and intimate social relatedness. These elements combined can contribute to the formation and development of *group attachment*, as conceptualised by Bowlby [3].

Group members present themselves with many different symptoms and problems, but also carry with them a wealth of experience and a capacity for supporting one another, as well as other strengths that can be used therapeutically in the group situation.

In the Bionian model, the analyst is paradoxically the sole (*leaderless*) group leader, and becomes the *only* source of higher-level functioning, interpretation and knowledge. In the Foulkesian model, the conductor is *not* the sole group leader, but takes the lead in enabling members to eventually constitute themselves in a *group of co-therapists* [31].

A group-analytic conductor is meant to foster not so much frustration, but tolerance and appreciation of individual differences—a real challenge in its own right. This distinct attitude is an effective way of encouraging members to participate actively in their own therapeutic process. Sometimes, but by no means always, such a conductor allows the group to cast him or her in the role of *leader*.

As the group matures through reliance on its own strength, the conductor or therapist's role evolves from being a leader *of* the group to becoming a leader *in* the group: the *authority* of the conductor is integrated into the *authority* of the group [5].

Group Analysis is not psychoanalysis of the group as if it were a *quasi-individual* [17, 18, 25] or individual analysis in the group [47], but therapy *of* the group, *by* itself, including its members and the conductor [23].

Bion and Foulkes were on common ground in their recognition of an unconscious mind, with transference defence mechanisms, both in the individual and in the group. With that said, Foulkes also gave himself permission to become a *member* of the group and introduced a new frame of reference, in which the transference develops in a different way due to its multi-personal distribution [28].

Some group analysts have attempted to integrate both approaches [2, 5, 20, 28, 48, 49]. But these attempts at working towards a rapprochement of the Tavistock and group-analytic models have been an exception to the norm. The reality is that neither Bion nor Foulkes (or their followers) appeared to significantly influence each other, although they both approached group therapy from the perspective of the group as-a-whole.

Certainly, there has been more emphasis on the differences between the two theories and subsequent clinical modalities. By the time Foulkes came to group psychotherapy, he was an experienced psychoanalyst and saw the group as a set of individuals whose interactions and communication became his focus. In contrast to that, when Bion approached group therapy, his experience was in a large organisation (the British Army) and he focussed on the group as an entity in itself. Hence,

> *Foulkes applied individual psychology to groups; Bion applied organisational psychology to groups. ([49], p. 353)*

In attachment terms, we may say that, in the traditional Tavistock model, it is more difficult for members to perceive the group as a *secure base*, although they are confronted more openly with group transference interpretations, particularly regarding possible manifestations of their unconscious hostility.

In contrast, in the group-analytic model, there is more room for the exploration of multiple aspects of the transference, including transferences of individual members to the therapist or conductor, as well as transferences amongst members themselves.

Optimally, the so-called *group matrix* can become a *secure base* for the patient to explore safely.

Nevertheless, it is striking that, in his many publications, Foulkes hardly referred to attachment or human development. In fact, the words development or attachment do not appear in any of the indexes of his books.

These terms are also absent in the index of *The Practice of Group Analysis* [50]. This book, with contributions from early generations of group analysts, is still largely considered a blueprint of group-analytic psychotherapy.

Consequently, in the thinking, training and practice of group analysts, past and present, there has been a concerning absence of attachment-based thinking, with only a few exceptions [5, 12, 30, 43, 44, 51–54].

Fortunately, in the last two decades, other clinicians and researches have contributed to the study of attachment into the field of group psychotherapy, particularly in North America and in Europe.

In this sense, we would like to direct the reader towards the work of McCluskey [55, 56], Flores [57], Markin and Marmarosh [58], Page [59], Marmarosh et al. [60], Marmarosh and Tasca [61], Marmarosh [45, 62, 63], Tasca [64], Wajda and Makara-Studzińska [65, 66], Tasca and Maxwell [46].

We may say that, in different ways, these authors have postulated that there is a group attachment system which, based on evolution, predisposes humans to seek security and form bonds with social groups, in addition to the dyadic or interpersonal attachment system. Although these two attachment systems (dyadic and group) are different, in many ways they overlap, have important similarities, and influence and complement each other [5].

Our own view is that person-to-person attachment and person-to-group attachment represent two relatively independent but interconnected domains. In order to further investigate and understand the nature of group attachment, it is essential to identify what exactly people are attached to when they interact *in* the group and *with* the group, not only with group members or leaders, but also with the group as-a-whole.

In fact, one of us had put across a tentative definition of this important concept, which tries to integrate group analysis with attachment-based thinking. Of course, this description can be revised and improved as further research moves along:

> *Group attachment can be conceived as a construct that brings together a complex constellation of significant attachment relationships, in the group and with the group;*

> *that is, with its members, with its leaders and with the group as-a-whole, in order to maximise survival, protection, development, creativity and full realisation of human capabilities, as a person and as a species. [67].*

6. Conclusion

The group is a deeply humanising entity with healing properties, and so can be a therapeutic and attachment space. In our evolution as a species, the group became an adaptive social organisation in the service of survival—a theme that has been at the front, in the origins of group therapy.

In fact, having to fight and survive two world wars had a strong bearing in the genesis and development of the two main models of group psychotherapy in Great Britain, those of Bion and Foulkes. Despite their differences, these approaches can be integrated and complement each other.

Certainly, no individual, however isolated in time and space, should be regarded as outside a group or lacking in multiple manifestations of group lives, including group attachment, as formulated by Bowlby in 1969 and further investigated by a number of authors, particularly in North America and Europe, in recent decades.

Group attachment is highly relevant to group psychotherapy; studying its nature and therapeutic implications should be an integral part of the training of psychotherapists and other mental health professionals across the board, especially those working with groups.

In an appropriate group climate, patients can perceive their therapy group as an attachment figure.

Author details

Arturo Ezquerro[1]* and María Cañete[2]

1 International Attachment Network and Institute of Group Analysis, London, UK

2 Institute of Group Analysis, London, UK

*Address all correspondence to: arturo.ezquerro@ntlworld.com

References

[1] Kaplan HI, Sadock BJ, editors. Comprehensive Group Psychotherapy. Baltimore, MA and London, UK: Williams & Wilkins; 1983

[2] Pines M. Circular Reflections: Selected Papers on Group Analysis and Psychoanalysis. London: Jessica Kingsley; 1998

[3] Bowlby J. Attachment and Loss, Attachment (1991 edition). Vol. 1. London: Penguin Books; 1969

[4] Ettin MF. Foundations and Applications of Group Psychotherapy: A Sphere of Influence. Boston, MA: Allyn and Bacon; 1992

[5] Ezquerro A, Cañete M. Group Analysis Throughout the Life Cycle: Foulkes Revisited from a Group Attachment and Developmental Perspective. London: Routledge; 2023

[6] Jung C. Collected Works. Vol. 9. Princeton, NJ: Princeton University Press; 1969

[7] Hawkins D. Understanding reactions to group instability in psychotherapy. International Journal of Group Psychotherapy. 1986;**36**(2):241-260

[8] Hearts LE. The emergence of the mother in the group. Group Analysis. 1981;**14**(1):25-32

[9] Trist E. Working with Bion in the 1940s: The Group Decade. In: Pines M, editor. Bion and Group Psychotherapy. London: Routledge; 1992. pp. 1-46

[10] Bion WR. The Long Week-End 1897-1919: Part of Life. Abingdon, UK: Fleetwood Press; 1982

[11] Dicks HV. Fifty Years of the Tavistock Clinic. London: Routledge & Kegan Paul; 1970

[12] Ezquerro A. Encounters with John Bowlby: Tales of Attachment. London: Routledge; 2017

[13] Bion WR. The leaderless group project. Bulletin of the Menninger Clinic. 1946;**10**:77-81

[14] Bion WR, Rickman J. Intra-group tensions in therapy. The Lancet. 1943;**2**:678-681

[15] Ezriel HA. A psychoanalytic approach to group treatment. British Journal of Medical Psychology. 1950;**23**:59-74

[16] Ezriel HA. Notes on psychoanalytic group therapy. Psychiatry. 1952;**15**:119-126

[17] Ezriel HA. The role of transference in psychoanalytic and other approaches to group treatment. Acta Psychotherapy. 1959;**7**(suppl):101-116

[18] Sutherland J. Notes on psychodynamic group therapy. Psychiatry. 1952;**15**:111-117

[19] Malan DH, Balfour FH, Hood VG, Shooter AM. Group psychotherapy: A long-term follow-up study. Archives of General Psychiatry. 1976;**33**(11):1303-1315

[20] Garland C, editor. The Groups Book. Psychoanalytic Group Therapy: Principles and Practice. London: Karnac; 2010

[21] Foulkes SH. Group analysis in a military neurosis centre. Lancet. 1946;**1**:303-313

[22] Foulkes SH. Introduction to Group Analytic Psychotherapy. London: Heinemann; 1948

[23] Foulkes SH. Therapeutic Group Analysis. London: George Allen & Unwin; 1964

[24] Foulkes SH. Group Analytic Psychotherapy: Method and Principles. London: Gordon & Breach; 1975

[25] Bion WR. Experiences in Groups. London: Tavistock; 1961

[26] Freud S. Group Psychology and the Analysis of the Ego, Standard Edition of the Complete Works of Sigmund Freud, (1953 edition). Vol. 18. London: Hogarth Press; 1921

[27] Ezquerro A (2004a) El grupo en la clínica. Primera parte: Aspectos históricos. En Caparrós N (ed) Y el Grupo Creó al Hombre. Madrid: Biblioteca Nueva, pp. 193-211.

[28] Ezquerro A. The Tavistock and group-analytic approaches to group psychotherapy: A trainee's perspective. Psychoanalytic Psychotherapy. 1996;**10**(2):155-170

[29] Ezquerro A (2004b) El grupo en la clínica. Segunda parte: Enfoques grupo-analíticos. En Caparrós N (ed) Y el Grupo Creó al Hombre. Madrid: Biblioteca Nueva, pp. 212-227.

[30] Ezquerro A. Apego y desarrollo a lo largo de la vida: El Poder del Apego Grupal. Madrid: Editorial Sentir; 2023

[31] Ezquerro A. Group psychotherapy with the pre-elderly. Group Analysis. 1989;**22**(3):299-308

[32] Blackwell D. Psychotherapy, politics and trauma: Working with survivors of torture and organized violence. Group Analysis. 2005;**38**(2):307-323

[33] Hopper E. The Social Unconscious: Selected Papers. London: Jessica Kingsley; 2003

[34] Holmes J. John Bowlby and Attachment Theory. London: Routledge; 1993

[35] Bowlby J. The study and reduction of group tensions in the family. Human Relations. 1949;**2**:123-128

[36] Bowlby J. The role of the psychotherapist's personal resources in the treatment situation. Bulletin of the British Psychoanalytical Society. 1991;**27**(11):26-30

[37] Bowlby J. Maternal Care and Mental Health. Geneva, Switzerland: World Health Organization; 1951

[38] Bowlby J. Child Care and the Growth of Love. Harmondsworth, UK: Penguin Books; 1953

[39] Bowlby J. The nature of the child's tie to his mother. International Journal of Psychoanalysis. 1958;**39**:350-373

[40] Bowlby J. Attachment and Loss, Separation, Anxiety and Anger (1991 edition). Vol. Vol 2. London: Penguin Books; 1973

[41] Bowlby J. Attachment and Loss, Loss, Sadness and Depression (1991 edition). Vol. Vol 3. London: Penguin Books; 1980

[42] Cañete M, Ezquerro A. Bipolar affective disorders and group analysis. Group Analysis. 2012;**45**(2):203-217

[43] Ezquerro A (1991) Attachment and its circumstances: Does it relate to group analysis? [Theoretical dissertation for membership of the Institute of Group

Analysis (IGA)]. Archives IGA Library, London

[44] Glenn L. Attachment theory and group analysis: The group matrix as a secure base. Group Analysis. 1987;**20**(2):109-126

[45] Marmarosh CL, editor. Attachment in Group Psychotherapy. New York: Routledge; 2020

[46] Tasca GA, Maxwell H. Attachment and group psychotherapy: Applications to work groups and teams. In: Parks CD, Tasca GA, editors. The Psychology of Groups: The Intersection of Social Psychology and Psychotherapy Research. New York: American Psychological Association; 2021. pp. 149-167

[47] Burrow T. A Search for Man's Sanity: Selected Letters with Biographical Notes. New York: Oxford University Press; 1958

[48] Brown D. Bion and Foulkes: Basic assumptions and beyond. In: Pines M, editor. Bion and Group Therapy. London: Routledge; 1992. pp. 192-219

[49] Hinshelwood RD. Bion and Foulkes: The group-as-a-whole. Group Analysis. 2007;**40**(3):344-356

[50] Roberts J, Pines M, editors. The Practice of Group Analysis. London: Routledge; 1991

[51] Adshead G. Psychiatric staff as attachment figures. British Journal of Psychiatry. 1998;**172**:64-69

[52] Maratos J. Self through attachment and attachment through self in group therapy. Group Analysis. 1996;**29**(2):191-198

[53] Marrone M. Attachment and Interaction. London: Jessica Kingsley; 1998

[54] Zulueta F. From Pain to Violence: The Traumatic Roots of Destructiveness. London: Whurr; 1993

[55] McCluskey U. The dynamics of attachment and systems-centred group psychotherapy. Group Dynamics: Theory, Research, and Practice. 2002;**6**:131-142

[56] McCluskey U. A model of group psychotherapy based on extended attachment theory: A preliminary report. Irish Association of Humanistic and Integrative Psychotherapy. 2007;**52**:71-81

[57] Flores PJ. Group psychotherapy and neuro-plasticity: An attachment theory perspective. International Journal of Group Psychotherapy. 2010;**60**(4):546-570

[58] Markin RD, Marmarosh CL. Application of adult attachment theory to group member transference and the group therapy process. Psychotherapy: Theory, Research, Practice, Training. 2010;**47**(1):111-121

[59] Page TF. Applications of attachment theory to group interventions: A secure base in adulthood. In: Bennett S, Nelson JK, editors. Adult Attachment in Clinical Social Work. New York: Springer; 2010. pp. 173-191

[60] Marmarosh CL, Markin RD, Spiegel E. Attachment in Group Psychotherapy. Washington, DC: American Psychological Association; 2013

[61] Marmarosh CL, Tasca GA. Adult attachment anxiety: Using group therapy to promote change. Journal of Clinical Psychology. 2013;**69**(11):1172-1182

[62] Marmarosh CL. Empirical research on attachment in group psychotherapy:

Moving the field forward. Psychotherapy. 2014;**51**(1):88-92

[63] Marmarosh CL. Attachment in group psychotherapy: Bridging theories, research and clinical technique. International Journal of Group Psychotherapy. 2017;**67**(2):157-160

[64] Tasca G. Attachment and group psychotherapy: Introduction to a special section. Psychotherapy. 2014;**51**(1):53-56

[65] Wajda Z, Makara-Studzińska M. Attachment in group psychotherapy. Part 1: Theoretical aspects. Psychoterapia. 2018a;**186**(3):7-17

[66] Wajda Z, Makara-Studzińska M. Attachment in group psychotherapy. Part 2: Empirical research. Psychoterapia. 2018b;**187**(4):57-67

[67] Ezquerro A (2019) The power of group attachment. Group Analysis North Open Seminar, University of Manchester, UK

Section 2

Children and Yoga

Chapter 3

Benefits of Yoga on Children

Mei-Ling Lin

Abstract

This chapter begins with an introduction of yoga and available yoga programs or curriculum for children of all ages and all abilities. Next, it summarizes the theoretical frameworks that support the investigation of the benefits of yoga, with an emphasis on the sensory integration theory. Third, this chapter draws on empirical studies from multiple disciplines to pinpoint the physical, mental, and social benefits of yoga on children with and without special needs. To conclude this chapter, case examples are utilized to showcase the implementation of yoga activities in school and group settings. Suggestions for researchers and practitioners who work with children are discussed as well.

Keywords: yoga, sensory integration, children, health benefits, well-being

1. Introduction

Yoga is a mind-body practice that originated in ancient India and has been gaining popularity worldwide due to its numerous physical, mental, cognitive, and spiritual health benefits [1]. While practicing yoga, individuals are instructed to focus their attention on their body posture, breathing, emotional awareness, and meditation [2]. In recent years, yoga has become increasingly popular in children and youth populations. Yoga programs designed for young learners often incorporate storytelling, games, music, and imagination to make the yoga practice fun and engaging. See **Table 1** for a listing of children's yoga programs that are available in the United States.

2. Conceptualizing the benefits of yoga from sensory integration theory perspectives

The sensory integration (SI) theory and the definition of sensory integration (SI) were formulated by Dr. Jean Ayres as "the neurological process that organizes sensations from one's own body and from the environment" (p. 11) [4]. Individuals learn knowledge and skills by reading, listening, speaking, and writing or manipulating [5]. The SI theory postulates that learning, or adaptive behaviors, is dependent on the ability to process and integrate sensation and use it to regulate emotions and plan movements. Practicing yoga, from the perspectives of the SI theory, is a learning process; competently and safely performing yoga is viewed as an adaptive behavior. See **Figure 1** for a schematic representation of practicing yoga based on the SI theory.

Curriculum/ program	Brief description	Recommended age range
Yoga Calm (https:// www.yogacalm.org/)	• Combines yoga poses with breathing techniques, games, storytelling, and relaxation techniques to develop physical, social emotional, and cognitive skills. • Beneficial for children with attention and social difficulties.	Ages 6–10 years
Yoga Ed (https:// yogaed.com/)	• Provides more than 450 mindful activities, yoga, and educational resources to promote physical health, emotional regulation, and academic success in children.	Online classes for all ages; subscription is needed
Little Flower Yoga (https://www. littlefloweryoga.com/)	• Their school wellness project teaches mindfulness practices, relaxation techniques, breathing, and yoga poses aiming to enhance emotional regulation, stress management, and academic learning.	PreK & K-12 students. In-person in NY & online classes.
Yogarilla (https:// www.superduperinc. com/yogarilla.html) [3]	• A card deck that consists of 55 cards, each featuring a different yoga pose and illustrations on how to perform the pose. Ideas on how to adjust or modify each yoga pose to accommodate the child's special needs are provided. • The cards are color-coded by difficulty level and can be used to create custom sequences and routines tailored to the abilities of individual children.	Children of all ages

Table 1.
Children's yoga program and curriculum in the United States.

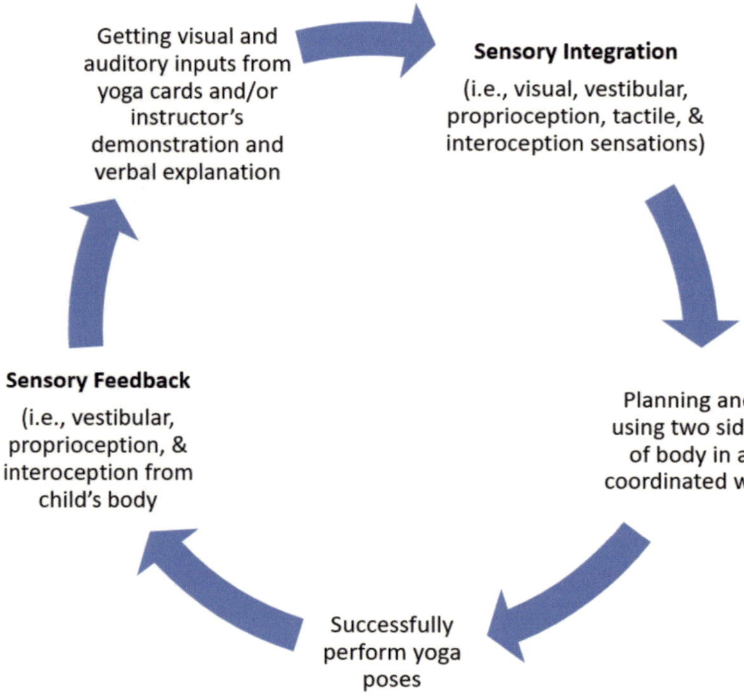

Figure 1.
A schematic representation of practicing yoga based on the SI theory. Adapted from Figure 1-1 A schematic representation of the learning component of SI theory [6].

While practicing yoga, a child is presented with visual information about certain yoga poses from cards/pictures or from yoga instructor's demonstration. The instructor may supplement their demonstration with verbal explanations or guided imagination (auditory information). To follow and successfully perform the yoga poses, the child then integrates the visual and auditory inputs with their ability to plan and use two aides of their body in a coordinated way, their ability to form the spatial relationship of different body parts in their mind (i.e., body scheme), and their ability to sense the internal signal from their body to breath. According to the SI theory, the bilateral coordination skills, body scheme, and breathing are hypothesized to be rooted in individual's vestibular, proprioception, tactile, and interoception processing abilities [6].

Notably, when a child is trying to imitate and perform yoga poses, he/she is obtaining sensory feedback from their body and their surrounding environment, specifically, the feedback from their body about their head position and balance (vestibular), the spatial relationship of different body parts (proprioception), and their breath (interoception). The feedback from their surrounding environment may include, but not limited to visual, auditory and tactile inputs (e.g., touching a yoga ball). The SI theory also postulates that the sensory feedback generated in the context of a just right postural or movement challenge contributes to improved sensory integration/processing, thereby enhancing learning and adaptive behavior [6].

So, upheld by the SI theory, the benefits of yoga may be contributed directly by the sensory feedback the child's body obtains during the practice of yoga and improved sensory processing following the practice of yoga. Proprioception is defined as perception or awareness of the position and movement of the body [7]. In the neuroscience literature, proprioceptive feedback, obtained from proprioceptive receptors located in muscle spindles and joints, have been clinically observed to have a calming effect [8–10]. This may explain the emotional or psychological benefits associated with practicing yoga. The vestibular system enables the perception of balance and provides information about body position, facilitating quick compensatory movements in response to both internally initiated and externally applied forces [11]. Together, vestibular and proprioceptive processing contribute to the coordination of head and body movement in space, the development of bilateral coordination, and the development of postural control (e.g., equilibrium). This may explain the physical health benefits of practicing yoga. Also, both proprioceptive and vestibular inputs have been linked to increased arousal levels [12]. This may explain the cognitive benefits (i.e., attention and learning readiness) of practicing yoga. The mental, physical, and cognitive benefits of yoga practices jointly contribute to an individual's self-awareness and social interaction with other people at different developmental stages.

3. Understanding the benefits of yoga for children from scientific evidence

Since yoga is considered a mind-body practice and often embedded in mindfulness practices and mindfulness-based interventions, and the deep breathing technique is an integral part of yoga practices, the findings from empirical studies that investigate the effects derived from deep breathing techniques as well as mindfulness and yoga practices are summarized in the following.

The previous research findings have revealed that instructing third- and fifth-grade students to engage in deep breathing techniques prior to tests led to reduced test anxiety and enhanced test performance [13, 14].

Mindfulness practice involves cultivating a state of heightened awareness attained through nonjudgmental attention to the present moment [15]. Across adolescent, adult, and geriatric populations, mindfulness practice has demonstrated associations with a range of benefits encompassing interpersonal aspects (such as fostering healthy relationships), emotional well-being (including decreased loneliness, stress, and anxiety), as well as intrapersonal advantages (such as the development of empathy, compassion, self-efficacy, attention, and executive functioning) [16–21]. Systematic reviews and meta-analyses conducted on mindfulness-based interventions implemented in school settings have established a positive correlation between mindfulness practices and enhanced mental health outcomes. These outcomes include reductions in stress, anxiety, and depression, as well as improvements in attention [22, 23].

Yoga offers numerous benefits for children with all abilities. Research has indicated that engaging in yoga serves as an effective intervention in mitigating anxiety, depression, and associated symptoms or behaviors among children and adolescents [24–26]. For typically developing children, yoga can also promote physical and mental health [27], as well as improve emotional regulation and self-awareness [28–30]. The study conducted by Morena-Gomez and Cejudo on kindergarten students revealed further advantages of mindfulness-based programs, which encompassed practices such as meditation, mandalas, and body awareness activities. These programs were found to contribute positively to overall child development, nonverbal development, and visual perception, while concurrently reducing maladaptive behaviors [31]. The above evidence support the use of mindfulness-based programs and yoga to enhance children's confidence, self-esteem, and social skills, while also providing an outlet for creativity and self-expression.

For children with special needs, yoga practices can help improve motor coordination, increase strength and flexibility, reduce anxiety and stress, and enhance overall well-being. For example, children and adolescents diagnosed with attention-deficit hyperactivity disorder (ADHD) have demonstrated improved attention and social behaviors following the participation in the mindfulness-based interventions (including yoga) [32]. Additionally, yoga has shown promise as a potential strategy for reducing stress and anxiety, enhancing quality of life, and improving lung function in children and adolescents diagnosed with asthma [33]. Moreover, a multicomponent program that involves yoga, dance, and modified relaxation response program has showed promising outcomes in improving behavioral and some core features of autism spectrum disorders for children aged 3–16 years [34]. Overall, there is gaining evidence to support the incorporation of yoga in treating children and adolescents with depression, sleep disorders, and as an augmentation therapy for pediatric populations with schizophrenia and ADHD [35].

4. Methods

Given the health benefits associated with yoga and mindfulness practices, the author conducted a needs assessment and developed a school-based mental health promotion program to address children's mental health needs in a US-Mexico border community. In this section, the community's mental health needs are presented first. Then, the group-based program activities are described in greater detail. Third, the lessons learned from program implementations are discussed; future directions for yoga research and practices are presented.

DOI: http://dx.doi.org/10.5772/intechopen.112105

4.1 Mental health needs in schools at the US-Mexico border community

School-age children living in an US-Mexico border city are facing multiple stressors in their school and home lives. In the state of Texas, third-grade to twelfth-grade students need to take the State of Texas Assessments of Academic Readiness (STAAR) test every spring semester. The increasing level of academic stress derived from numerous practice tests, quizzes, and exams in preparation for the STAAR test is noticeable and sensible. At the time of the needs assessment, no social emotional learning (SEL) curriculum was formally taught to students to recognize their own and others' emotions and to use stress management techniques to positively face and deal with stress and anxiety.

Notably, the elementary school served 535 students in kindergarten through sixth grade, predominantly children living in Hispanic families (92%) with low socioeconomic conditions (78%). Stressors associated with disadvantaged living conditions, along with stressors unique to the Hispanic population, such as language barriers, perceived discrimination, mental health stigma, and higher risks of having inconsistent health insurance coverage and unmet mental and behavioral needs, all indicate a need to improve mental health awareness, literacy, and access in this population [36].

To respond to the school's mental health needs, occupational therapy faculty and students from the University of Texas at El Paso collaborated with the school team to develop and pilot-test a "Tools for stress" workshop to lay the foundation for developing a school-wide mental health promotion program for the elementary school. The author's intention is multi-faced, including equipping elementary school students with evidence-supported coping strategies to address stress and anxiety, documenting scientific evidence to support the implementation of school-based mental health promotion programs, and establishing long-term university-school collaborative relationships.

4.2 Case 1: "Tools for Stress" workshop

"Tools for Stress," a 45-minute workshop for kindergarten through fourth-grade students (N = 382), was designed to fit into the school's career day schedule in which the speakers from the community come to speak their job or profession and answer students' questions. There were four classes per grade level, and each class had around 20 students [37].[1] On the date the workshop is held, each grade level would come into the school gymnasium that was set up to accommodate all the program activities. The workshop opened with questions such as, "what is stress?" and "how do you feel and what do you do when you are stressed?" to survey and further students' understanding of physical, emotional, and behavioral signs of stress. Onsite translation support was provided for non-English learners. The sequence of program activities all in a group format is presented in **Table 2**.

This workshop concluded with an anonymous survey to gain student's feedback (e.g., "how much did you like the activities?" and "how confident would you be to use the activities the next time you feel stress?"). Overall, this program obtained an overwhelming positive response from students. Of 364 valid surveys collected from participating students, 85% liked the yoga and deep breathing exercises, 95% liked the sensory bottle they made, and 82% indicated they were confident and competent about using the calming strategies in the future when feeling stressed. The school

---

[1] The fifth and sixth graders had schedule conflicts that precluded their inclusion.

Activity sequence	Description
1. Sensory bottle (20 minutes)	• Each student was given a clear bottle prefilled halfway with water to build their own sensory bottle. The student chose a "calming color" from various colors of glitter and/or food coloring to add to their bottle. The student then added clear glue to fill the other half of the bottle, and the bottle was tightly sealed. • Sensory bottle is used as a visual aid to help students shift their attention from stressful events to the present moment (watching the glitter settle until the bottle became clear again) [22, 38].
2. Deep breathing (5 minutes)	• The belly breathing and star breathing techniques were introduced. In a seated position, students were instructed to place one hand on their heart and the other hand on their belly and guided to "make your belly as big as a balloon" as they inhaled, then exhaled. Next, students received instructions to extend their fingers on one hand, resembling a star, and were guided to inhale as they used the pointer finger of their other hand to trace a path up the thumb and across each finger. They were then instructed to pause momentarily before exhaling while tracing down each finger [13, 31].
3. Yoga (10 minutes)	• Students learned and practiced balance poses, dynamic stretching, and free movements, coupled with deep breathing and soothing music [25, 31]. • A script wrote by a yoga instructor is used (see Appendix).

Table 2.
The "Tools for Stress" workshop overview.

counselor has continued to reinforce the strategies introduced in the workshop with students in 1:1 counseling session. However, the counselor also mentioned challenges to incorporate yoga and other mindfulness-based strategies into each classroom and an already-packed school daily schedule. The school administration requested that this program be continued and expanded for both students and teachers and broadened to include workshops for families.

4.3 Case 2: The school-wide mental health promotion program

In the fall of 2019, based on the feedback collected from the "Tools for Stress" workshop and the synthesis of scientific literature, occupational therapy faculty and students from UT-El Paso design a mental health promotion program and conduct an empirical study to explore its outcome on fifth and sixth graders' perceived ability to handle negative emotions (i.e., emotional self-efficacy, ESE) and their perceived levels of satisfaction with the program. This program consists of four in-person instructional sessions that integrate the existing evidence and incorporate specific lessons from the Zones of Regulation curriculum [39]. Every session was carefully planned to have a duration of 45 minutes and took place once a month within the school's indoor gymnasium during the physical education (PE) class time. The sessions were facilitated by second-year OT students, closely supervised by three OT faculty members, along with the participation of the school counselor and the school nurse. See **Table 3** for the program overview.

Results obtained from a sample of 100 students (39 boys and 60 girls, with 1 case of missing data; 57 fifth graders and 43 sixth graders) indicate that, for the entire group, there are no statistically significant differences in emotional self-efficacy (ESE) ratings before and immediately after the implementation of the mental health promotion program ($t(84) = -1.08$, $p = .29$). However, noteworthy findings emerge when examining the pretest and posttest scores. Students with lower ESE ratings before the program demonstrated improved ESE ratings after program participation ($t(46) = -3.258$, $p = .00$), while those with higher initial ESE ratings experienced a decline in ESE ratings ($t(37) = 1.98$, $p = .06$). No significant differences were observed between boys and girls or between fifth and sixth graders regarding ESE ratings before and after program implementation. Overall, more than 60% of the program participants expressed a neutral to positive attitude toward the program activities. Among all the program activities, students favored mandala coloring the most, followed by slime making, deep breathing, and yoga, respectively. Approximately 70% of the program participants expressed feeling both competent and confident in utilizing one of the calming tools they had learned during the program when facing future stress.

4.4 Discussion

Suggestions are made based on the two case examples for researchers and practitioners who consider implementing yoga programs or curriculum to address the social emotional needs of school-age children.

First, the collaboration among parents, teachers, and mental health providers (e.g., counselors, psychologists, and occupational therapists) is the key to the successful program implementation and the most optimal children outcome. Outside of the "Tools for Stress" workshop, the OT faculty set a booth at the school health fair to provide educational materials to increase parental awareness of family

Session # and topic	Session content
1. Knowing Stress and Emotions	• Introduce Zones of Regulation through handouts, a YouTube video, and examples prepared by instructors. • Categorize facial expression pictures into the most appropriate zone on a Zones of Regulation poster.
2. Exploring Calming Tools: Part I	• Mindful art: slime making; the use of slime as a fidget to shift their attention from stressful things to the object manipulation and de-stress is discussed. • Deep breathing technique: star breathing. • Mindful yoga: using cards that show the sitting and standing postures in the Yogarilla curriculum [3]. Students are guided to focus on their breathing, body postures, and movements during yoga practices.
3. Exploring Calming Tools: Part II	• Mindful art: mandala coloring. Students are instructed to focus on the mandala pattern, the color they want to use, and the strokes they make. • Deep breathing technique: "Lazy 8" breathing. Students are given instructions to follow the sequence of inhaling, pausing, and exhaling while tracing the horizontal depiction of the number eight on the provided handout. • Mindful yoga: utilizing cards that depict standing balance postures, which are considered more challenging in the Yogarilla curriculum [3]. The focus on breathing, body postures, and movements is emphasized.
4. Knowing When to Use Calming Tools	• Review the calming tools learned. • The Zones Tools worksheet that maps the calming tools with four zones of emotions. • The Zones Across the Day worksheet that allows students to visually examine the changes of their emotions during a day and pinpoint when they feel stressed, what they did when feeling stressed, how long they feel stressed, and what things they do to reduce stress.

Table 3.
Mental health promotion program overview [40].

mental health and to facilitate healthy ways to manage stress using the tools and strategies their child learned from the workshop. For teachers and paraprofessionals, two 1-hour workshops introduced evidence-informed stress management techniques (i.e., breathing exercises, yoga stretches, using a sensory board that included various textures) that could be implemented in the classroom to support students' self-regulation and address students' emotional and behavioral challenges. Under the circumstance that all the stakeholders are aware of the importance and benefits of yoga, children can be given provided numerous opportunities to practice yoga. And the benefits of yoga can be maximized and carried over to different environments.

Second, the timing of yoga instruction should allow students to immediately apply their learning to real-life situations. A comparison of the workshop satisfaction survey results and the research study's program satisfaction survey results showed that 85% of kindergarten to fourth-grade students like yoga and deep breathing. Yet only 27% of and 40% of fifth and sixth graders like yoga and deep breathing correspondingly. Additionally, the satisfaction ratings of the workshop activities were higher among younger elementary school students compared to the satisfaction levels of fifth and sixth graders in the implemented program. One possible reason for this disparity in the satisfaction survey outcomes is that younger students could immediately perceive the benefits of the calming tools they learned when they took the STAAR test. In contrast, older students completed the survey during the fall semester when no STAAR testing was conducted, which could explain their relatively lower satisfaction levels.

Third, early introduction of yoga and cultivation of child's interest in yoga are recommended. It is observed that younger students demonstrated better response and acceptance toward yoga and other program activities compared to older students. The developmental stage of middle childhood is characterized by the emergence of self-autonomy and a significant influence of peers within social networks. That is, older elementary school-age children may be more susceptible to peer pressure compared to their younger counterparts. As a result, they may be more inclined to mimic their peers' responses to stress and anxiety rather than adopting the strategies and techniques taught by adults. Since the motivation and the interest to learn yoga is the foundation for the continuation of practicing yoga, the future design of yoga programs or curriculum should shed more emphasis on early childhood populations.

Last but not the least, the integration of technology into yoga instruction and learning holds great potential for both practitioners and researchers. Utilizing web- or mobile-based applications, such as *Adventures in Emotional Literacy* developed for elementary school students (3C Institute, n.d.), offers the advantage of flexibility in terms of time and location to students to acquire emotional literacy and coping skills. This approach allows instructors to maximize in-person teaching time and to enable students to put into practice the knowledge and skills acquired through the e-curriculum. Gathering information such as program satisfaction, frequency of application use, and knowledge gained before and after program implementation can be easily achieved through web-based platforms and learning management systems.

5. Conclusion

To conclude this chapter, key information is highlighted as follows.

- Yoga is a mind-body practice; given the advance in current technology, the yoga programs designed for young learners are more accessible and are limited to in-person instruction.

- Using the sensory integration theory as the conceptual framework to study the benefits of yoga practices is an innovative perspective and needs more empirical support.

- Yoga is a valuable tool for promoting holistic development and well-being in children of all abilities. They can help children develop body awareness, improve flexibility and strength, reduce stress and anxiety, and cultivate mindfulness and self-awareness.

- It is of author's hope that the two cases examples, both are author's experience of using yoga and other mindfulness activities in an elementary school, will generate more discussions on feasible ways to use yoga in group therapies or formats.

Acknowledgements

I want to express my sincere gratitude to the UTEP College of Health Science, Occupational Therapy Program, faculty, and Classes of 2019 and 2020 students for the participation and ongoing support to this research project. I also want to acknowledge the REL Washington Elementary in El Paso, Texas, for their enthusiasm and dedication to this collaborative project and school mental health.

Conflict of interest

The author declares no conflict of interest.

Appendices and nomenclature

See sample yoga script.

A. Sample yoga script

Stand tall like a mountain (mountain will be the resetting posture/resting pose)—feet firmly planted down on the ground, arms out, palms out, strong finger reaching to the ground.

Breathing in and out of your nose—as your belly goes in and out. Mindful breathing as you breathe in for 1, 2, 3 and out 1-5.

Relax your arms out to the side—shrug your shoulders toward your ears as you breathe in and away from your ears as you breathe out of your mouth (loud audible) release and relax your shoulders (3×'s)

Roll your head in circles to the R

Roll your head in circles to the L

Now move around however feels good, stretching out your neck and relaxing your shoulders-freestyle while feet are firmly planted on the ground (if you feel silly, you can wiggle it out, if you feel tired, you can move nice and slow)

Come back to mountain, come back to a calm, slow breath. (Sometimes if you have a bad day, it's good to plant your feet firmly on the ground and take a few deep breaths)

Slowly bring your hands to your heart, bring your elbows out to your side, palms facing each other. Press your hands as hard as you can for 1, 2, 3 and relax (3x's)

Relax your arms down at your side, shake it out

Come back to mountain, stand tall and strong like a mountain, and take 3 deep breaths (guided), see how still you can be...

Now bring your arms out to your side, lift them up overhead like you're reaching for the sun/sky.

When your arms and hands are up in the sky, interlace your fingers and make a 'steeple', 'water gin' ...etc. Relax the shoulders down and reach your steeple up.

Because you are explorers, bend your knees a little bit and shoot up (jump) like a rocket ship.

Stand tall, take a deep breath in and reach to the L

Come back to center, bend your knees a little bit and shoot up(jump) like a rocket ship (blast off into space one last time).

Release your arms, shake them out.

Widen your stance a little more, reach your arms out to the side and be a star-shine bright like the brilliant stars you are! Twist to the right and left, shooting your star around while keeping your legs firmly planted on the ground.

Relax your arms, bring your legs back together.

Stand firm on your L leg and lift your R leg up and back.

Now we are going to pretend we are trees, plant your L foot (leg) down and lift your R leg up to the inside of your L leg (above or below your knee)

Grow your tree, blow in the wind, etc.

Plant your R root (leg) down and lift your L leg up to the inside of your R leg (above or below your knee).

Grow your tree, blow in the wind, etc.

Release and shake it out.

Dancer- bring your R foot into your R hand behind you. Kick your R foot back into your R hand and reach forward with your L hand.

Come back to mountain and prepare to do the other side.

Bring your L foot into your L hand behind you. Kick your L foot back into your L hand and reach forward with your R hand.

Release, and shake it out.

Come back to mountain and take a deep breath in and exhale loudly.

Bring your hands to your waist, stand tall like a superhero. Bring your elbows back like you are trying to touch them together. Lift your chest, lift your heart, lift your head and be the strong, confident, unique superhero you know you are.

While in superhero—take three deep breaths in and out your nose.

Relax arms down at your side.

Bring your hands back to your heart and say, "I AM AWESOME."

Then turn to your friends and say, "YOU ARE AWESOME!"

Then we end our practice with, "The awesome in me recognizes the awesome in you! Namaste"

Author details

Mei-Ling Lin
The University of Texas Health Science Center at San Antonio, San Antonio, TX, USA

*Address all correspondence to: linm2@uthscsa.edu

References

[1] Smith BR. Body, mind and spirit? Towards an analysis of the practice of yoga. Body & Society. 2007;**13**(2):25-46

[2] McCall T. Yoga as Medicine: The Yogic Prescription for Health and Healing. New York City, New York, U.S.: Bantam; 2007

[3] Mielke K, Richmond M-L. Yogarilla® Exercise and Activities. Greenville, SC: Super Duper Publications; n.d.

[4] Ayers AJ. Sensory Integration and Learning Disorders. Los Angeles, CA: Western Psychological Services; 1972

[5] Berninger VW. Development of language by hand and its connections with language by ear, mouth, and eye. Topics in Language Disorders. 2000;**2000**:65-82

[6] Bundy AC, Lane SJ. Sensory integration: A. Jean Ayres' theory revisited. In: Bundy AC, Lane SJ, editors. Sensory Integration: Theory and Practice. 3rd ed. Philadelphia: F.A. DAVIS; 2020. pp. 2-21

[7] Bear M, Connors B, Paradiso MA. Neuroscience: Exploring the brain. In: Exploring the Brain. enhanced ed. Burlington, Massachusetts, U.S.: Jones & Bartlett Learning; 2020

[8] Chen H-Y, Yang H, Chi H-J, Chen H-M. Physiological effects of deep touch pressure on anxiety alleviation: The weighted blanket approach. Journal of Medical and Biological Engineering. 2013;**33**(5):463-470

[9] Reynolds S, Lane SJ, Mullen B. Effects of deep pressure stimulation on physiological arousal. The American Journal of Occupational Therapy. 2015;**69**(3) 6903350010p1-p5

[10] Vasa RA, Carroll LM, Nozzolillo AA, Mahajan R, Mazurek MO, Bennett AE, et al. A systematic review of treatments for anxiety in youth with autism spectrum disorders. Journal of Autism and Developmental Disorders. 2014;**44**:3215-3229

[11] Purves D, Augustine G, Fitzpatrick D, Katz L, LaMantia A, McNamara J, et al. The Vestibular System. Neuroscience. 2nd ed. Sunderland, MA: Sinauer Associates; 2001

[12] Rose MF, Ahmad KA, Thaller C, Zoghbi HY. Excitatory neurons of the proprioceptive, interoceptive, and arousal hindbrain networks share a developmental requirement for Math1. Proceedings of the National Academy of Sciences. 2009;**106**(52):22462-22467

[13] Khng KH. A better state-of-mind: Deep breathing reduces state anxiety and enhances test performance through regulating test cognitions in children. Cognition and Emotion. 2017;**31**(7):1502-1510

[14] Larson HA, El Ramahi MK, Conn SR, Estes LA, Ghibellini AB. Reducing test anxiety among third grade students through the implementation of relaxation techniques. Journal of School Counseling. 2010;**8**(19):n19

[15] Kabat-Zinn J. Mindfulness. Mindfulness. 2015;**6**(6):1481-1483

[16] Davis DM, Hayes JA. What are the benefits of mindfulness? A practice review of psychotherapy-related research. Psychotherapy. 2011;**48**(2):198

[17] Firth AM, Cavallini I, Sütterlin S, Lugo RG. Mindfulness and self-efficacy in pain perception, stress and academic

performance. The influence of mindfulness on cognitive processes. Psychology Research and Behavior Management. 2019;**2019**:565-574

[18] Gallegos AM, Lytle MC, Moynihan JA, Talbot NL. Mindfulness-based stress reduction to enhance psychological functioning and improve inflammatory biomarkers in trauma-exposed women: A pilot study. Psychological Trauma: Theory, Research, Practice, and Policy. 2015;**7**(6):525

[19] Jin Y, Zhang M, Wang Y, An J. The relationship between trait mindfulness, loneliness, regulatory emotional self-efficacy, and subjective well-being. Personality and Individual Differences. 2020;**154**:109650

[20] Schonert-Reichl KA, Lawlor MS. The effects of a mindfulness-based education program on pre- and early adolescents' well-being and social and emotional competence. Mindfulness. 2010;**1**(3):137-151

[21] Mak C, Whittingham K, Cunnington R, Boyd RN. Efficacy of mindfulness-based interventions for attention and executive function in children and adolescents—A systematic review. Mindfulness. 2018;**9**(1):59-78

[22] Carsley D, Khoury B, Heath NL. Effectiveness of mindfulness interventions for mental health in schools: A comprehensive meta-analysis. Mindfulness. 2018;**9**(3):693-707

[23] Klingbeil DA, Renshaw TL, Willenbrink JB, Copek RA, Chan KT, Haddock A, et al. Mindfulness-based interventions with youth: A comprehensive meta-analysis of group-design studies. Journal of School Psychology. 2017;**63**:77-103

[24] Hagins M, Haden SC, Daly LA. A randomized controlled trial on the effects of yoga on stress reactivity in 6th grade students. Evidence-Based Complementary and Alternative Medicine. 2013;**2013**:607134

[25] Weaver LL, Darragh AR. Systematic review of yoga interventions for anxiety reduction among children and adolescents. The American Journal of Occupational Therapy. 2015;**69**(6) 6906180070p1-p9

[26] James-Palmer A, Anderson EZ, Zucker L, Kofman Y, Daneault J-F. Yoga as an intervention for the reduction of symptoms of anxiety and depression in children and adolescents: A systematic review. Frontiers in Pediatrics. 2020;**8**:78

[27] Benavides S, Caballero J. Ashtanga yoga for children and adolescents for weight management and psychological well being: An uncontrolled open pilot study. Complementary Therapies in Clinical Practice. 2009;**15**(2):110-114

[28] Butzer B, LoRusso AM, Windsor R, Riley F, Frame K, Khalsa SBS, et al. A qualitative examination of yoga for middle school adolescents. Advances in School Mental Health Promotion. 2017;**10**(3):195-219

[29] Dariotis JK, Mirabal-Beltran R, Cluxton-Keller F, Gould LF, Greenberg MT, Mendelson T. A qualitative evaluation of student learning and skills use in a school-based mindfulness and yoga program. Mindfulness. 2016;7:76-89

[30] Bazzano AN, Sun Y, Zu Y, Fleckman JM, Blackson EA, Patel T, et al. Yoga and mindfulness for social-emotional development and resilience in 3-5 year-old children: Non-randomized, controlled intervention. Psychology Research and Behavior Management. 2023;**16**:109-118

[31] Moreno-Gómez A-J, Cejudo J. Effectiveness of a mindfulness-based social–emotional learning program on psychosocial adjustment and neuropsychological maturity in Kindergarten Children. Mindfulness. 2019;**10**(1):111-121

[32] Jensen PS, Kenny DT. The effects of yoga on the attention and behavior of boys with attention-deficit/hyperactivity disorder (ADHD). Journal of Attention Disorders. 2004;**7**(4):205-216

[33] Lack S, Brown R, Kinser PA. An integrative review of yoga and mindfulness-based approaches for children and adolescents with asthma. Journal of Pediatric Nursing. 2020;**52**:76-81

[34] Rosenblatt LE, Gorantla S, Torres JA, Yarmush RS, Rao S, Park ER, et al. Relaxation response–based yoga improves functioning in young children with autism: A pilot study. The Journal of Alternative and Complementary Medicine. 2011;**17**(11):1029-1035

[35] Balasubramaniam M, Telles S, Doraiswamy PM. Yoga on our minds: A systematic review of yoga for neuropsychiatric disorders. Frontiers in Psychiatry. 2013;**3**:117

[36] Perreira KM, Gotman N, Isasi CR, Arguelles W, Castañeda SF, Daviglus ML, et al. Mental health and exposure to the United States: Key correlates from the Hispanic community health study of Latinos. The Journal of Nervous and Mental Disease. 2015;**203**(9):670-678

[37] Lin M, Fierro C, Medrano C, Arroyos D, Medrano G. Addressing mental health needs of elementary school children through university-community collaboration. AJOT Special Interest Section Quarterly Practice Connections. 2020;**5**(3):20-22

[38] Worthen E. Sensory-based interventions in the general education classroom: A critical appraisal of the topic. Journal of Occupational Therapy, Schools, & Early Intervention. 2010;**3**(1):76-94

[39] Kuypers L. The Zones of Regulation. Minneapolis, MN: Think Social Publishing; 2011

[40] Lin M-L, Paat Y-F, Cooper A, Molina C, Smith E, Millar K, et al. A universal mental health promotion program that demonstrates psychosocial benefits for elementary school students who perceive low emotional self-efficacy. Journal of Occupational Therapy, Schools, & Early Intervention. 2022;**2022**:1-16

Section 3

Music Therapy

Chapter 4

Emotive Quality Transformations in Music: The Psychoaesthetics of Emotion Polarization

Tirtha Prasad Mukhopadhyay and Armando Perez

Abstract

The author investigates if musical modes have definitive emotive contents and following this, if certain modes have affective potentials that are targeted and specific to forms of appraisal. Do certain note clusters occupy emotive loops in accordance with certain basic emotion types - and so what may be, therefore, the general rule for valence appraisals of basic emotions activated by targeted note clusters. The co-existence of connectionist circuits or engram activation routes would have to be conjectured. Finally, a multidisciplinary approach shows us that a new pattern of a psychoaesthetic valence-aggrandized happy or positive version of emotions would have to be considered. There is no such existing proposal for a 'version' theory of basic emotions. We propose that a psychoaesthetic version of basic emotions exists. Next, we also defend the possibility of polarization of emotions through entrainment. Music may have the ability not just to evoke any given emotional state or state of feelings in the psychoaesthetic spectrum but also to polarize basic emotions to create a value-added experience. Conclusions from the discussion suggest that music appraisals may have far-reaching implications for the understanding of the ontological quality of music and its relations to well-being and mental health.

Keywords: basic emotion, emotion polarization, extra basic emotion, psychoaesthetics, music therapy

1. Introduction

Music consists of patterns of emoted vocal (or instrumental) sounds – as such it is a product of behavioral practice that arouses and appropriates feelings. These feelings are usually oriented toward appraisals of happy, felicitous, and positively energetic character [1, 2]. More philosophical proponents in the field of psychology and neuroscience opine that music has its origins in the neuro-ecological 'body–mind' continuum [3], which refers to the impulse from the environment inducing the specific sonic patterns which embody and modify human feelings [3, 4]. The literature also suggests that the sound [sonic] frequency at the base of musical articulation [a] already evolved ethologically as emotively understood modulation of audited frequencies [5, 6], and as such manifested itself through two possible axes: (i) namely, as a momentarily integrated 'note' with its expectancies and its recourse to episodic memory [7], and (ii) second, a sequence of notes (i.e. peaks or nodes of frequencies) creating temporal modulation or what we more commonly call 'progression', 'melody' or 'rhythm' indicative of the time game of musical performances [8]. Both processes ([a] i and [a] ii) help coopt formal elements from collectively intelligible expression or audition that occur within the context of any articulate culture. Anyone willing to arrive at the well-springs of music must feel this integrated moment that we call 'music' where the musical tendency is always inspiring human subjects to emote out states of pleasure through notes that combine in harmony, pleasure, and the energetic take on life.

Secondly, the consumer of music must find recourse and patience in this idea of music as a profoundly auditory expression or articulation of a sonic note, executed either in a series, and as an emission of notes such as generates an 'esthetic' category for a context of listeners [9–11]. Music emotion is esthetic emotion. Esthetics constitutes an area of psychological speculation which still crawls in its infancy. But recent studies on neurodynamic changes of 'core affect' better explains – how music emotions are manipulated through the system to elicit these specific types of esthetic-emotive states – what we may properly designate esthetically 'charged' (or polarized) emotive states. Henceforth, it should be logical to associate music emotions with esthetically satisfactory perceptions in emotion induction and appraisal rather than as a simplistic or 'primary' emotion consciousness [9, 10, 12–15]. A strong case for music emotions is made by Flaig and Large [9].

Entrainment is believed to be a cause of emotive triggers in experiences of musical harmony [16]. In general, however, the literature on musical emotions, with a few exceptions, reveals a lack of emphasis on cognitive appraisal of music effects, like that of esthetic arousal, etc. [17]. Indeed, there might be various types of music emotion – which indeed is what appears to be true from common sense observation, although here we are considering the possibility or overarching music emotion – 'esthetic music'. Could we set up standards of measurement for such themes [18–20].

Earlier observations on musical emotions lead to a fecund intellectual discussion on the necessity of recognizing first, the esthetic state elicited in the process, alone. This is tentatively articulated by Ekmann in his early inconclusive studies on esthetic emotions as Extra Basic Emotional State (henceforth EBES) – some of that foundation of a separable and hierarchically organized or vertical-integrative state gives way to explaining the moment of any esthetic emotional experience. Now, music is not compared to or assumed to be an 'esthetic' state per se, although it is one [21, 22]. As just mentioned, in consultation psychology, and in applied psychology in general "esthetics" has not been defined in the literature. First, esthetic emotions of a psychologically sound subject – are a kind of EBES, an extra basic emotion. Ekmann speaks of Basic Emotion types and hence external stimuli elicit basic emotions like anger, sadness, disgust, or happiness [12]. But esthetic emotions are not categorized within the ambit of Basic Human emotions. In the literature, psychologists have referred to emotions of "awe", "pleasant surprise", or "admiration" Ekman. Unfortunately, although all these characteristics define esthetic emotions, they are not able to explain the range and extent of esthetic emotions as a visible emotional state. Even as emotional states are considered to be reflexive conditions of the body, and thus as embodied cognitive behavioral perceptions, there is no embodied esthetics of the esthetic emotions - such as are elicited in theater, performances, movies, art galleries, or by the presence of art, or esthetically satisfactory installations – or especially, as discussed here. Levinson, Juslin and Slobodan and Juslin, Flaig and Large, Scherer, Scherer, and colleagues all do mention and bring music esthetics to the forefront of research.

Music emotion first then may be considered empirically as belonging to the incipiently identified category of EBESs [21]. Just as Ekman speaks of such undefined or uninvestigated properties of emotion such as 'admiration' 'awe' or 'surprise' it would be possible to add the effects of 'esthetic' sensations like 'thrill' or additional 'euphoria' or general sense of happy well-being (Moors and Kuppens 2008; Robinson 2008). These value-added EBESs are always rapidly guaranteed in experiences caused by musical performances. Secondly, EBES holds a special import for musical emotions as the latter comprise direct, unmediated provocations of lifting (esthetic) emotive states. The 'core affect' precept of a constructivist architecture of musical esthetics requires a similar assumption of the underlying natural or instinctive and inner propensities of emotions [13]. Again, Levinson [23] and Juslin [11, 12] recognize the basic emotion reflex framework from which esthetic emotions - such as especially musical emotions are found to evoke their effects for listeners. In the vocabulary, this is referred to as the BRECVEM method of explaining how musical emotions are evoked. The psychoaesthetics of music, if explained especially from a psychogenetic point of view, are also understood as based on neural activation of emotive circuits that hold episodic musical memories that create expectancies and retinues of convention – indeed all conjointly believed to be carrying and releasing musical emotions as their point of a destined output.

But this by no means assumes that these musical emotions are also being part of the experience afforded in terms of 'esthetic experiences' as well.

As stated by Juslin for example the proposed nine-fold architecture of the BRECVEM – or Brain Stem Reflex, Rhythmic Entrainment, Evaluative Conditioning, Contagion,

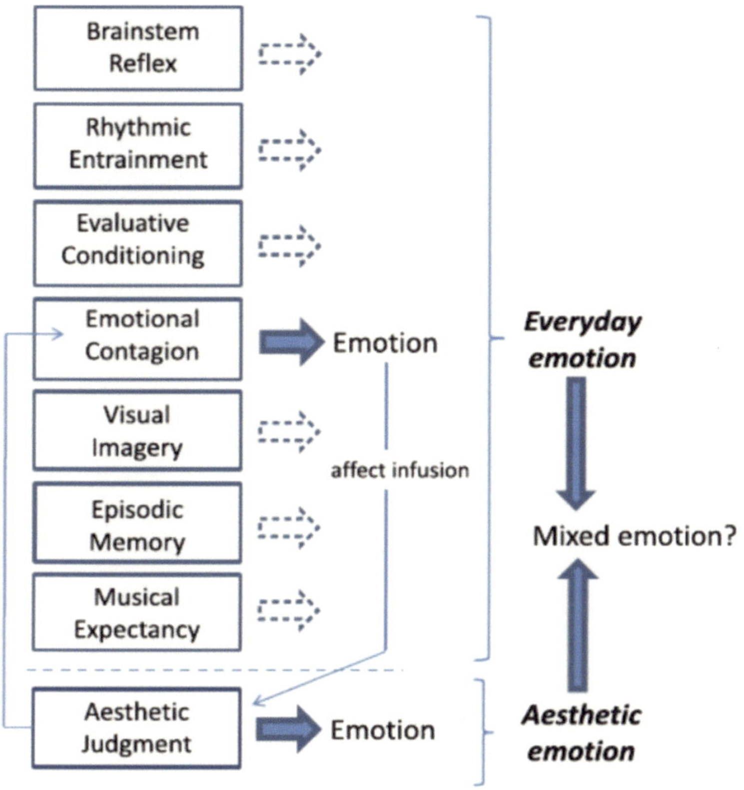

Figure 1.
Juslin's model of "esthetic" emotion elicitation through music (Juslin 2017).

Visual Imagery, Episodic Memory, Musical Expectancy, and Esthetic Judgment [21] enumerate these steps in the process of esthetic appraisal of music. But Juslin's conceptual framework of music emotion elicitation includes a reference to 'Esthetic Judgment' (See **Figure 1** following Juslin 2017 [11]). Music itself is considered as an emotive trigger or as Juslin calls it "Emotional responses ... [that] need to consider underlying mechanisms but it leads to an esthetic emotion which can blend or condition 'everyday emotion' as its appraisal mechanism" [24]. The point about aestheticity -deriving out of an assumed psychoaesthetic 'mechanism' (vide. **Figure 1**) of basic emotion materiality gives specificity and direction to questions arising in music emotions.

2. Musical affect leads us to believe more firmly in Esthetic emotions

Hence, music teaches us about the depth and power of esthetic emotions. Musical emotions are not just emotions - they refer to a specific way or polarization (**Figure 2**) which humans emote out within a range of musical affects. Sexual enhancement affect, dancing, physical emotions of release, and well-being are polarized toward vertical esthetic levels, of tranquilizing and more energy-arousing emotions. Levels must be recognized even in the case of musically evoked emotions [17]. The level change of energy [12, 14] or polarized happy feeling that is entrained in music elicitation must be recognized as inalienable element in the musical effect. Even if it were true that only a certain category of music was able to perform that kind of calming musical affective

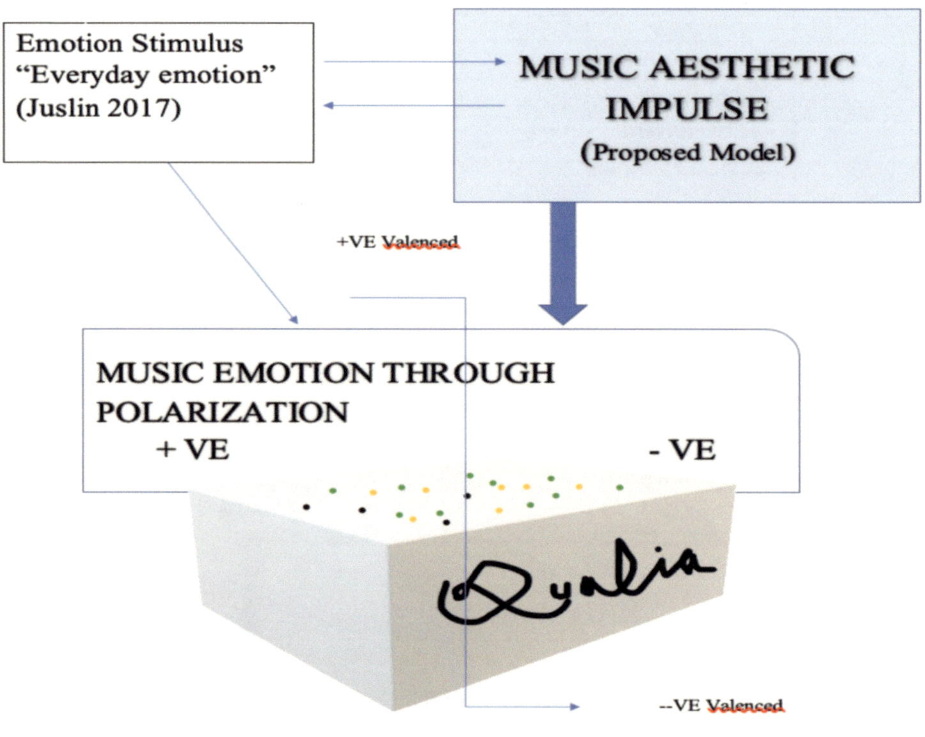

Figure 2.
Proposed model of transformation of emotive qualia through neural polarization-based thematically on Juslin [11]. Consider Juslin's model of "esthetic" emotion elicitation in the "MIXED EMOTIONS" state, which remains somewhat vague and indiscriminate.

DOI:http://dx.doi.org/10.5772/intechopen.110290

function. Yet music does it with the power and positive valence or charge - a degree of neural excitation that no other stimulus is able to provide.

3. The argument from intersectionality

Interdisciplinary methodology has the potential of demonstrating the complete circumplex trajectories of the emotion -of any emotion whatsoever but it appears to be more directly relevant for tracing the emotion extensions of emotions vis a vis emotion disorders. Any emotive condition or dysfunction is capable of being viewed through its affective other, or valence or alteredness: sad/happy; anger/tranquility, etc. I refer to the circumplex model only to suggest - as has been already considered in great detail by Frijda [25]. The studies of Frijda [25], have the most impressive till-date of basic documentation of what Frijda calls 'arousal'. Indeed, arousal is an indispensable factor in the evocation of emotions, including that of basic emotion states like that of fear or anxiety. Barrett also speaks of an architecture of arousal - the point is to note what I have suspected about emotions based on insights provided in traditions of emotion studies from very different philosophical or analytical traditions [26]. The same emotional traumas could be aroused and contemplated in a positive state of affects -so that the emotion or affect may harbor an intrinsic potential to transform and get aroused in a polarized manner. Valence is of the essence here and is directly related to the practice of polarizing emotive self-esteem, and in general, the ability to negotiate with negative tendencies, closedness, depression, and traumatic withdrawal [27].

The knowledge of these transforming valences of our physiologically built-in conditions (the EBESs) - the potential of emotive base change or neuronal replacement conditions are possibilities that remain to be labeled. Levitt asked in a very relevant manner: "Does the pattern of physiological reaction differs among emotional states; can these patterns be used to differentiate among the emotions?"

I believe that these are very important questions in the study of anxiety and fear - that is only being raised in a rather inchoate form in contemporary applied psychology and psychosocial behaviorism. They point to the need for a reconsideration of the basic emotion paradigm in psychology and to replace it with a basic circumplex emotions model which looks at emotion as its own medicine, and as a feeling that could be traumatized or impaired but then also cultivated to release and realize an altered, esthetically polarized, therapeutic level of normative well- being for itself.

The second question would be could emotive engrams actualize such esthetic trances? The proposition that certain emotions can undergo perceptual changes or alterations within the valence scale has not been extensively suggested. Musical emotions function in thematic musical variations of love songs, or music of love or yearning, music of desire, mating or union desiring musical moan are evident in popular love songs, articulate music, and instrumental melody that mime the desire or yearning or moaning provocations. If we were to consider the sad or love emotion in music alone, and in sibling art forms such as poetry: say in the songs of Widsith the far wanderer – the long peregrinatory yearning songs of a transcendental other – all even through variations in cross-cultural manifests of the archetypal love song – there is demonstrable truth of this assumption about the intrinsic emotive quality of the love song. The love qualia get propositionally visible, objectified, modulated, and appraised for emotive arousal and appraisal.

Hence, we might conjecture about the presence of a basic Ekmann emotional qualia (EBES) of the love song – it is a cross-cultural phenomenon and may also be identified under a certain emotive rubric of effects. The contention however is not related to whether a basic 'moan' or 'yearn' emotion is embodied and elected through music articulations of the love song. Certain aspects of this question are admittedly debatable -the fundamental assumption about the cross-cultural validity of basic musical emotions or types. Yet some rhythms are amenable or appraised as more sad emotional articulations and yet others as more comedic -these broad variations are evidently and obviously visible within the large gamut of desire moaning - as we are calling them here.

Extra Basic Musical EBES, may be similar to the distinctive component forms of the BRECVEM suggested by Juslin – that there is a sad to romantic range for the musical emotions of moaning or yearning love songs, or moaning calls. Could it be possible to review the neurodynamic or synaptic neurodynamism or neuroinhibitory history of these formations or qualia, at all? From a more speculative point of view - we could move toward a reconsideration of the qualitative characters of momentary feelings associated with a known or given musical emotion. The history of this research is indeed scarce and either egotistical or dismissive by virtue of exclusive philosophical stance-taking attitudes [21]. Juslin comes very close to stating the virtue of this question and yet his review of the literature turns out to be both falling out of focus [11]. He claims for example:

The psychological process through which this is achieved is referred to as 'the underlying mechanism'. A description of the psychological process should not be confused with its neural implementation in the brain or with the phenomenological experience it seeks to explain [24]. Yet there is no adequate selection of the reference to this underlying mechanism. His citation of Dennett here is also misleading – Dennett's speculative theorizing is based partly on personal observations with its lack of comprehensive and rounded analysis and its default assumption of cognitive categories that do not refer to emotion at all [28].

4. Do Esthetic engrams exist?

Thus, we may ask: What are the underlying emotional causes of the music emotions of moaning songs? More interestingly and fundamentally however we may ask how we could describe this "underlying mechanism" hypothesis of the musical emotions. Unless this description is available, we may not be able to suggest why music emotions like that of the love song with its objectification of the moaning call - the 'desire-feeling' evoked in love situations may be mixed or modulated with EBES-like moments of admiration, gratitude, awe, surprise, thrill and above all euphoria. A love song's melody, despite its variations, will need to have a core affect proposition at its neurodynamic level, one that remains a core affect for the performer as well as the cultural participant of that music – and is, as such capable of being accessible to entrained episodic memory, as part of the paradigmatic engram at the CNS and ANS circuits of the given emotion. But that is not enough – there is very little literature or studies to guide us here. Unless we define and amplify the science of psychoaesthetic states the core affect proposal for exclusive esthetic types of emotions may fall apart.

A brief review of the literature on neurodynamic oscillations reveals that there is very limited hypothesis testing in the field of experiments on psychoaesthetic modularity. Unfortunately, as a review article Wagemans's summary assessment of psychoaesthetics [29]. Does not consider the art experience as a primarily emotional experience. But as objects mensurated in terms of symmetry and matching, to pre-existing models. It may be worth noting from Wagemans is with reference to Zajonc. As far as emotive experience making and consumption are concerned it is with Zajonc that we begin to compile the timeline for an adequate understanding of the emotive component [30]. Preferential emotional seeking is close to the heart of the question that also relates to musical appraisal. Here we shall refer strictly to music emotion causation. In traditional psychological approaches to musical emotions, or more properly speaking to the causal factors of music emotions, Levinson takes a lead role in defining what Levinson calls the "music moment" [28]. Levinson is however drawing attention to the structural architectures, and responses elicited by musical expectations. Levinson's findings found support for the review assessments of Slobodan and Juslin [18] and Juslin [11]. Some very concrete help in this regard comes from neuropsychologists who have located and correlated the functions of amygdala to specific emotional reflexes elicited by music- Gosselin and colleagues have shown amygdala activation and impairment correlations to music emotions in the amygdala -and the independence of brain circuits for emotions from brain circuits that may be responsible for valence and arousal [31]. Zajonc and Panskepp's pioneering research in neuroscience has enabled neuropsychologists to develop a clearer picture of emotion activation by means of music -and hence indeed music is incontrovertibly considered as an emotion tool for several levels of experiment in brain circuit projections [32, 33].

5. Could engram's sources be conditioned or qualified?

Last but not the least, we should have to conclude with insights we have derived from a brief review of the approaches. The broad indications in the psychoaesthetic definition of music are as follows:

A. Levinson and Juslin's methods of psychological appraisal structures including the BRECVEMA deconstruction of the component methods of musical appraisals [11, 23]

B. The structural approach to psychoaesthetics and emotions as it appears in Wagemans and colleagues [29]

C. Lesion analysis methods with also specific findings from investigations of impairment and responses (of the amygdala and midbrain) to musical emotions and appraisal processes such as that of Gosselin and colleagues [31, 34].

These three outlines in psychology, neuropsychology, and neuro-psychological lesion analysis impairment inferences suggest at least three important notions.

Musical emotions are engendered through the activation of engrams in the amygdala but findings such as Fritz and colleagues [22] and Gosselin [31] suggest that the amygdala does not itself impair valence function in music emotional appraisal architectures. If the valence is considered important - at least in positivizing – basic emotion experiences (EBESs) through music, then the co-existence of other circuits or engram activation routes would have to be conjectured [33, 35]. Finally, therefore the emphasis on a multidisciplinary approach as in Scherer and Coutinho [36] and Cochrane and colleagues [1] show us, the pattern of a psychoaesthetic valence-aggrandized happy or positive version of emotions would have to be considered. There is no such proposal for a version theory of emotions – as is possibly proposed in a psychoaesthetic approach which defends a theory of polarization of emotions through entrainment. Music may have the ability not just to evoke any given emotional state or state of feelings but also polarize itself to create a value-added experience. In that case, the neural architecture of music evocation must be revised. The lesion impairment methods could lead the way into this kind of investigation of the polarization or version theory of emotional alteration for which musically transformed representations of emotions remain strong evidence. The version-handling power of music implies a change of valence and positive polarization, such as the kind of energy state that anticipates satisfaction, gratefulness, admiration, and above all a sense of fulfillment that turns into well-being and relief from stresses of daily life. This signifies a search into the realm of psychoaesthetics where music helps in understanding precisely how multiple factors may be involved in a singular emotive appraisal.

6. Conclusions

In conclusion, we may attempt to explain the 'underlying causality' or 'underlying mechanism' that demonstrates how music emotions are generated in the scheme of environmental interactions of the human being, the one which creates humans like music emoters. Whether neurodynamic modularity is worth identifying may be justified by the fact that at least on the one physiological level embodied emotions reveal that changes in emotional quality are already self-evident perceptions – the mere corporeal entity remains a metaphor of the process which is mooted. The human body models emotive qualia both in its elicitatory trajectory as well as in its effects of change. The body may change in its expression of a certain primary emotion like anger or sadness, yet the same emotional symbols may be enjoyed in the subject's body with mediated tonal peak, as, in an opera or recital. The entire organism finds its polarized otherness through the amygdala and the autonomous nervous system. It is only more than plausible that the same changes are wrought at the synaptic level, along with the retrieval of episodic memory through functional inhibitors. A spatial diagram of such synaptic polarization, as in **Figure 2**, should resemble a map of chemical responses on the ionic level. On every level emotive transformation of the same emotional impulse, the change in the character of qualia, and the induction of a specific or altered mood state following a change in the musical provocation, must all be understood as a fundamental dynamic quality of emotions circumplex.

DOI:http://dx.doi.org/10.5772/intechopen.110290

Author details

Tirtha Prasad Mukhopadhyay* and Armando Perez
University of Guanajuato, Salamanca, Mexico

*Address all correspondence to: tirtha@ugto.mx

References

[1] Cochrane T, Fantini B, Scherer KR. The Emotional Power of Music: Multidisciplinary Perspectives on Musical Arousal, Expression, and Social Control. Oxford: OUP; 2013

[2] Gomez P, Danuser B. Relationships between musical structure and psychophysiological measures of emotion. Emotion. 2007;7(2):377. DOI:10.1037/1528-3542.7.2.377

[3] Edelman GM, Tononi G. Consciousness: How Matter Becomes Imagination. UK: Penguin; 2013

[4] Clarke EF. Lost and found in music: Music, consciousness and subjectivity. Musicae Scientiae. 2014;**18**(3):354-368. DOI:10.1177/1029864914533812

[5] Alcorta CS, Sosis R, Finkel D. Ritual harmony: Toward an evolutionary theory of music. Behavioral and Brain Sciences. 2008;**31**(5):576-577. DOI:10.1017/S0140525X08005311

[6] Boero DL, Bottoni L. Why we experience musical emotions: Intrinsic musicality in an evolutionary perspective. Behavioral and Brain Sciences. 2008;**31**(5):585-586. DOI:10.1017/S0140525X08005396

[7] Large EW, Kim JC, Flaig NK, Bharucha JJ, Krumhansl CL. A neurodynamic account of musical tonality. Music Perception: An Interdisciplinary Journal. 2016;**33**(3):319-331

[8] Large EW. A dynamical systems approach to musical tonality. Nonlinear Dynamics in Human Behavior. 2011;**2011**:193-211

[9] Flaig NK, Large EW. What is special about musical emotion? Physics of Life Reviews. 2013;**10**(3):267-268. DOI:10.1016/j.plrev.2013.07.014

[10] Scherer KR, Schorr A, Johnstone T, editors. Appraisal processes in emotion: Theory, methods, research. New York: Oxford University Press; 2001

[11] Juslin PN. From everyday emotions to aesthetic emotions: Towards a unified theory of musical emotions. Physics of Life Reviews. 2013;**10**(3):235-266. DOI:10.1016/j.plrev.2013.05.008

[12] Huron D. Theories, frameworks and aesthetics comment on "from everyday emotions to aesthetic emotions: Towards a unified theory of musical emotions" by Patrik Juslin. Physics of Life Reviews. 2013;**10**(3):271-272

[13] Flaig NK, Large EW. Dynamic musical communication of core affect. Frontiers in Psychology. 2014;**5**:72. DOI:10.3389/fpsyg.2014.00072

[14] Grandjean D, Sander D, Scherer KR. Conscious emotional experience emerges as a function of multilevel, appraisal-driven response synchronization. Consciousness and Cognition. 2008;**17**(2):484-495. DOI:10.1016/j.concog.2008.03.019

[15] Penman J, Becker J. Religious Ecstatics, "Deep Listeners," and Musical Emotion. Review Literature and Arts of the Americas, 2009;**4**(2):49-70

[16] Scherer KR, Zentner MR, Schacht A. Emotional states generated by music: An exploratory study of music experts. Musicae Scientiae. 2001;**5**(1):149-171

[17] Moors A, Kuppens P. Distinguishing between two types of musical emotions and reconsidering the role of appraisal. Behavioral and Brain Sciences. 2008;**31**(5):588. DOI:10.1017/S0140525X08005438

[18] Sloboda JA, Juslin PN. Psychological Perspectives on Music and Emotion: Music and Emotion: Theory and Research. Oxford: OUP; 2011

[19] Watson KB. The nature and measurement of musical meanings. Psychological Monographs. 1942;**54**(2):i. DOI:10.1037/h0093496

[20] Witvliet CC. The impact of music-prompted emotional valence and arousal on self-report, autonomic, facial EMG, and startle responses across experimental contexts (Doctoral dissertation, ProQuest Information & Learning)

[21] Ekman P. Basic emotions. Handbook of Cognition and Emotion. 1999;**98**(45-60):16

[22] Fritz T, Jentschke S, Gosselin N, Sammler D, Peretz I, Turner R, et al. Universal recognition of three basic emotions in music. Current Biology. 2009;**19**(7):573-576. DOI:10.1016/j.cub.2009.02.058

[23] Levinson J. On the concept of music. In: Aesthetics. New York: Routledge; 2017. pp. 192-195

[24] Juslin PN, Västfjäll D. Emotional responses to music: The need to consider underlying mechanisms. Behavioral and Brain Sciences. 2008;**31**(5):559-621. DOI:10.1017/S0140525X08005293

[25] Frijda NH. The place of appraisal in emotion. Cognition & Emotion. 1993;7(3-4):357-387

[26] Barrett LF. Discrete emotions or dimensions? The role of valence focus and arousal focus. Cognition & Emotion. 1998;**12**(4):579-599. DOI:10.1080/026999398379574

[27] Kuppens P, Tuerlinckx F, Russell JA, Barrett LF. The relation between valence and arousal in subjective experience. Psychological Bulletin. 2013;**139**(4):917. DOI:10.1037/a0030811

[28] Dennett DC. The evolution of culture. The Monist. 2001;**84**(3):305-324

[29] Wagemans J. Towards a new kind of experimental psycho-aesthetics? Reflections on the Parallellepipeda project. i-Perception. 2011;**2**(6):648-678. DOI:10.1068/i0464

[30] Zajonc RB. Feeling and thinking: Preferences need no inferences. American Psychologist. 1980;**35**(2):151. DOI:10.1037/0003-066X.35.2.151

[31] Gosselin N, Peretz I, Johnsen E, Adolphs R. Amygdala damage impairs emotion recognition from music. Neuropsychologia. 2007;**45**(2):236-244. DOI:10.1016/j.neuropsychologia.2006.07.012

[32] Panksepp J. The emotional sources of" chills" induced by music. Music Perception. 1995;**13**(2):171-207. DOI:10.2307/40285693

[33] Peretz I, Gagnon L, Bouchard B. Music and emotion: Perceptual determinants, immediacy, and isolation after brain damage. Cognition. 1998;**68**(2):111-141

[34] Koelsch S, Fritz T, Cramon DY, Müller K, Friederici AD. Investigating emotion with music: An fMRI study. Human Brain Mapping. 2006;**27**(3):239-250. DOI:10.1002/hbm.20180

[35] LeDoux JE. Emotion circuits in the brain. Annual Review of Neuroscience. 2000;**23**(1):155-184. DOI:10.1146/annurev.neuro.23.1.155

[36] Scherer KR, Coutinho E. How music creates emotion: A multifactorial process approach. The Emotional Power of Music: Multidisciplinary Perspectives on Musical Arousal, Expression, and Social Control. 2013;**18**:121-145

Chapter 5

Music and Its Healing Effects

Songül Mollaoğlu and Mukadder Mollaoğlu

Abstract

Music therapy, which is widely recommended for patients living with chronic problems, is actually a mind-body therapy. This therapy, which has been used clinically for more than a century, is one of the oldest treatment methods and is known to have been used in the treatment of patients in various cultures for four thousand years. Music therapy, known as simple harmonic movement, is rich in psychological and physiological effects. Used to support emotional, mental, and physical health, music therapy is an integrative art therapy method that provides a way to express feelings and experiences that cannot easily be expressed through words. Particularly in recent years, it has been observed that interest in traditional and complementary medicine in the field of health has increased worldwide. In this context, music therapy, one of the art therapy methods, attracts attention as a treatment method preferred by people among medical alternative treatment methods. In this section, the journey of music therapy from past to present and the neurophysiology of music are briefly explained and its effects on health problems are discussed in the light of findings in the literature.

Keywords: music therapy, healing effect of music, history of music therapy, physiology of music, integrative art therapy

1. Introduction

The word musica is taken from the Greek "mousike" or "mousa". Nine fairy girls, who were considered the daughters of Zeus, the greatest god of the Greeks, were called "mousa" (mus). The ancient Greeks believed that these fairy girls were responsible for organizing the beauty and harmony of the whole world. It is accepted that the word music, which exists in almost all languages today, is derived from the root "muz" [1].

With the existence of medicine, music therapy has also existed. When we look at the use of music in medicine throughout history, it is seen that this association has always existed and continues until today. In ancient times, music was more common in belief-based use regarding the human soul. It is stated that the history of music therapy dates back to primitive tribes. According to the belief in primitive tribes, every being had its own voice and song. It was thought that the sound and song that a person would react to would be found by a sorcerer and the evil spirits inside him would be removed in this way and the cure would be cured. In addition, according to primitive tribes, diseases were caused by evil spirits and demons, and their treatment was done by a respected person called a shaman. According to mythology, Shamans would remove evil spirits from the patient's body with rhythm and dance accompanied by music. In Christianity, church leaders used music as a treatment for mental illnesses [2, 3].

Apollo was a god believed to have played the lyre beautifully in ancient Greek mythology. He was considered the god of medicine. According to the belief in mythology, the music needed to relieve people's troubles and give them joy was performed by playing the lyre [4]. It is said that Orphee, one of Apollo's sons, played the lyre very well. In ancient Greece, mathematician and philosopher Pythagoras also played the lyre. After Pythagoras, the basic thought and moral teachings of the classical Greek music movement developed with Plato and Aristotle [4, 5].

While Aesculape used the trumpet to treat deafness, Homera is known to have used music in surgeries and demonstrated its effectiveness. Plato stated in 400 BC that music gives tolerance and comfort to the individual by affecting the depths of the soul with harmony and rhythm [6]. Egyptians used music during childbirth to reduce labor pain. In ancient Rome, Celcus and Areteus pointed out that music soothes the soul and is good for mental illnesses. It is reported that Confucius talked about the positive effects of music on people, that it calmed people and had beneficial effects on blood circulation [7].

In the late twentieth century, music therapy studies made significant progress, especially in the West. In the examinations, these studies appear as non-clinical studies as well as clinical studies. It is seen that music therapy in an experimental sense is also used in qualitative and quantitative research and is used especially to improve the physical and psychological conditions of patients during and after medical procedures [8]. Thomas Edison's invention of the phonograph in 1877 and his development of the disc recorder in 1886 were the beginning of the use of music in patient treatment in hospitals. As a result, music has been used in hospitals for therapeutic purposes since the first half of the twentieth century. The first studies were mostly conducted on anesthesia and analgesia applications. In the mid-twentieth century, researchers began to develop theories about the neurological basis of the effects of music and experimentally investigated the effects of music on physiological parameters [6, 9].

One of the first doctors who wanted to make music therapy available clinically was French neurologist Philipe Pinel. Pinel, who bases his studies on mental health on understanding people and advocates humanistic treatment methods, is known to advocate the use of music in treatment [4]. Dr. Willer Van der Wall took the first step in working on music therapy in America. In 1920, he conducted some research on music in hospitals and prisons in Pennsylvania and New York states and determined that music had positive contributions to people and had soothing and positive stimulating effects. The practice of music therapy as a profession was started during World War I. Music was used in hospitals to heal traumatic soldiers injured in war and to relieve their pain psychologically. Music therapy, which was accepted as a branch of science in America in 1977, has been used as an effective method in psychiatric diseases since the 1950s [10, 11].

The aim of music therapy studies that started in the hospital is to keep patients as involved in life as possible, to make them productive, to enable them to socialize, and to increase their adaptation to daily life. Art therapy by providing inter-institutional cooperation: It is a mental health specialty that uses the creative process in art to increase and improve the physical, mental, and emotional well-being of individuals of all ages [12].

This process, followed by music as a therapy method, has been used as an integral part of the field of music and health throughout human history. Today, music therapy, as a form of expression that helps people express their emotions and reflect their unconscious emotions, adds meaningfulness to people's inner world. Today, music therapy has become a form of help sought for various reasons such as coping with the symptoms of chronic diseases, reducing the side effects of medications, strengthening the immune system, preventing mental depression, strengthening healthy behaviors, and preventing tension and loss of strength.

2. Physiology of music

Music therapy has a history of thousands of years and today it emerges as a globally accepted field of expertise. The relationship between music and therapy goes back a long way. In fact, it is one of the oldest treatment methods. It is said that it is used in different cultures and civilizations. Music, one of the art therapy methods, appeals to the feelings and thoughts of the living being. Music has its own elements. There are expression elements such as genre, structure, rhythm, and language. For music therapy purposes, musical features such as rhythm, harmony, and melody are used [6, 13].

In the last 20–25 years, music, many studies have been conducted on its effects on neurotransmitters, hormones, cytokines, lymphocytes, vital signs, and immunoglobulins. Especially in the last decade, there has been an increasing number of studies examining the psychological and neurological effects of music on patients and the benefits of music on health [10].

Music is a unique stimulus because it causes both physiological and psychological responses in the listening individual. Music therapy, known as simple harmonic movement, is rich in psychological and physiological effects. When there is an auditory stimulus force, it is perceived as moving in a series. It begins with the compression of air molecules in the external ear canal, reaches the tympanic membrane, and finally passes through the cochlea to reach the nerves in the somatosensory region. Music stimulation leads to psychobiological improvements in this pathway. This way creates many effects on the person who listens to music (**Figure 1**) [14, 15]. Listening to music affects the autonomic nervous system and serves a healing function by causing relaxation in the organism. The first place where the sound of music is perceived is the auditory center located in the temporal lobe of the brain. Music perceived in the auditory center stimulates the thalamus, medulla, hypothalamus, midbrain, and pons [14, 16]. Music that affects different areas of the brain can reduce pain, for example, by causing the release of endorphins and enkephalin. As a result of its effect on the right hemisphere of the brain, it causes some effects on the limbic system and psychophysiological reactions occur, creating a therapeutic effect. Brain waves can be accelerated or slowed down by music, and it has an anxiolytic effect by helping to coordinate muscle tension and movements. As the pressure on neurotransmitters in the center increases, mood changes are achieved and anxiety decreases by correcting the nerves in the medulla oblongata [14–16].

As mentioned above, music creates a therapeutic effect by affecting the autonomic nervous system and neuroendocrinal activities. As it is known, the center of emotions is the limbic system. The influence of emotions on the limbic system is also related to the fact that the music reaching the body is not loud and has a normal tone and pitch. Thus, music listened to in a normal tone can transform negative emotions or disturbing emotions into positive emotions in the limbic system [17, 18]. As a result of a series of neuroendocrinological activities and autonomic processes stimulated by the effect of music in the organism, differences in emotions and physiological parameters occur in individuals. The parasympathetic nervous system takes action, slowing down and

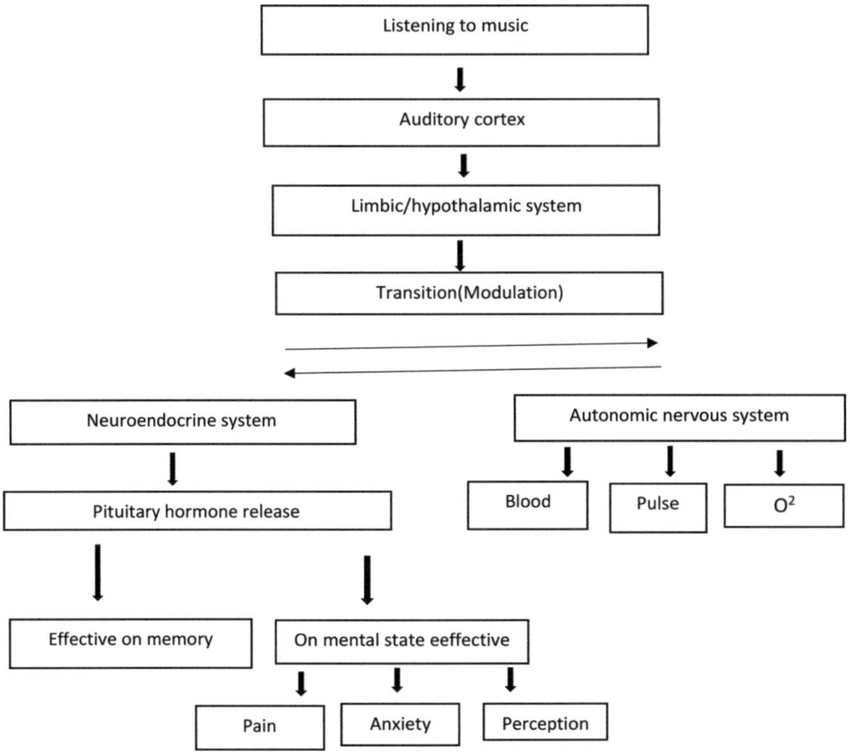

Figure 1.
Physiological mechanism of music therapy [14].

improving vital signs, especially breathing, blood pressure, and pulse. On the other hand, the pituitary gland, activated by the neuroendocrinological effect, accelerates the release of endorphin. Endorphins both regulate the mood in the organism and reveal the therapeutic effect of music through its natural pain-relieving effect, thus reducing both pain and anxiety levels in those who listen to music. It also enables people to perceive difficult situations more positively [18, 19].

Research conducted so far indicates that the effect of music on immune response and psychological and neurological diseases is due to its important effect on stress pathways. Studies on the subject have determined that there is a significant relationship, especially between music and dopamine, adrenaline, testosterone, and serotonin. These hormones, which affect the emotional state of the organism, have a positive effect on people who listen to music. Considering the relationship of these hormones with psychiatric diseases, it is known that music therapy is widely used especially in this field [6, 10]. Physiological effects of music therapy ranges from reducing psychophysiological stress, pain, anxiety, and isolation to inducing a change in behavior and altering mood. Research has shown a significant relationship between music therapy and pain and anxiety. In addition to other neurohormonal effects, music therapy has many benefits for the organism, such as reducing nausea and vomiting due to chemotherapy, reducing anxiety, and pain, improving sleep quality in people with sleep problems, and increasing the comfort of the person by distracting attention. As we mentioned before, music also has benefits in regulating pulse, respiration, body temperature, and blood pressure due to its effect on the autonomic nervous system [10, 20].

Thus, music therapy has been actively used in healthcare environments as a result of the stages it has gone through from past to present. With the development of modern medicine, it is now used as an alternative and complementary method to relieve the symptoms of diseases along with medical treatment. Below, the effects of music on some symptoms are discussed, using the physiological effects of music on humans.

3. Pain - anxiety and music

Pain is defined by the Taxonomy Committee of the International Association for the Study of Pain as “an unwanted emotional sensation or behavioral pattern related to the individual’s past experiences, originating from a specific area of the body, whether or not due to tissue damage” [21, 22]. It is thought that the positive effect of music on pain management is that it affects the autonomic nervous system and increases the release of endorphins, resulting in less pain perception. It is stated that music therapy, which has a very long history, has come to the fore again in recent years with the increasing interest in non-pharmacological methods [22, 23].

The process of neurophysiology of music and its effect on humans, the transmission of music, begins with the compression of air molecules in the external ear canal, reaches the tympanic membrane and finally passes through the cochlea and reaches the nerves in the somatosensory region. It is sent to the hearing area of the brain by nerve cells. The transmitted musical stimulus is first pushed upwards in the part of the brainstem called the lateral lemniscus. In the brainstem, music is first evaluated and analyzed. Music perceived by the temporal lobe, the hearing center, causes stimulation in the thalamus, medulla, hypothalamus, midbrain, and pons. The thalamus decides the state of music within the brain. The influence of the thalamus is important for the evaluation of musical information. The first cortex regions provide hearing and analysis is done from the temporal lobe, the thalamus receives this information, sends it to the relevant areas in the brain and the music spreads in an area. Thus, the right hemisphere works on the progression of the music, the left hemisphere makes the appropriate analysis [24, 25].

Music affects the right hemisphere of the brain, causes psychophysiological responses through the limbic system, and causes the release of enkephalin and endorphins, resulting in a decrease in the level of pain. Brain waves can be accelerated or slowed down by music, and it has an anxiolytic effect by helping to coordinate muscle tension and movements. As the pressure on neurotransmitters in the center increases, mood changes are achieved and anxiety decreases by rehabilitating the nerves in the medulla oblongata [25]. Music causes both physiological and psychological responses in the individual who listens to it. The individual is more influenced by the music of his own culture. Because they can establish healthier communication with the music of their own culture. Individuals’ understanding of music varies depending on the social and cultural structure of the society they live in and the education they have received [25, 26].

Studies conducted in different clinical settings report that music therapy is an effective intervention method, especially for intensive care patients. In Elliot’s study in 1994, the effects of music therapy on anxiety, pain, and muscle relaxation were examined in patients hospitalized in the coronary intensive care unit with a diagnosis of ischemic heart disease. The study revealed that music had a positive effect on these patients and increased their comfort, and the importance of music as a therapy method was emphasized [27]. A similar study was conducted by Bolwerk. In this study, in patients with myocardial infarction in intensive care, it has been found that music is effective in reducing patients' pain and anxiety [28]. In another study, music therapy was used for the first time to reduce the pain and anxiety experienced by patients in the coronary intensive care unit and to increase the comfort of the patients [29]. Sullivan, in his study on patients hospitalized in coronary and surgical intensive care units, the patients listened to classical music, and it was determined that the patients' pain and anxiety decreased after music therapy [30]. Tse et al. in their study with experimental and control groups, investigated the effects of music therapy after nose surgery on postoperative pain, pulse, blood pressure, and analgesic use. They applied 30-minutes of music therapy to the experimental group patients intermittently for the first 24-hours after surgery and measured pain values 4 times during the intervention. As a result of the study, they showed that the pain level decreased significantly over time in the experimental group compared to the control group [31]. In their study with experimental and control groups, Allred et al. investigated the effect of music on postoperative pain. They randomly divided 56 patients who had knee replacement surgery into two groups. As a result of the study, they found that the pain averages of the patients in the experimental group decreased statistically significantly [32].

In a randomized controlled study conducted by Takmak et al. patients diagnosed with COVID-19 were listened to nature-based music, and its effect on stress, some physiological parameters, and adaptation to the prone position was evaluated. Accordingly, in the intervention group listening to music, the stress level decreased the oxygen saturation of the intervention group increased, and the time lying face down increased, compared to the control group. At the end of the study, the researchers concluded that listening to nature-based music in the prone position may reduce anxiety, increase adaptation to the prone position, and improve oxygenation and heart rate in conscious patients with hypoxemic respiratory failure [33].

In another study (2020), it was found that music therapy reduced the pain, anxiety, and depression levels of patients [13]. Music reduces muscle tension and affects the biological rhythm of individuals by causing brain waves to accelerate and slow down, affecting the parasympathetic nervous system, and increasing the release of endorphins [34, 35]. Chlan examined the effect of music on anxiety in patients receiving ventilator support and found that there was a decrease in the respiratory and pulse values of the patients in the music group [36].

4. Nausea-vomiting and music

Nausea and vomiting are common due to chemotherapy. Chemotherapy-related nausea and vomiting are the most common and serious side effects caused by chemotherapeutics. This is a common symptom in those receiving chemotherapy, and patients are very afraid of developing nausea and vomiting. It is recommended that music therapy be used in conjunction with other non-pharmacological methods to prevent chemotherapy-related nausea and vomiting. When the literature is examined, it is seen that many studies on music have been conducted with patients who have undergone bone marrow transplantation or solid organ transplantation, and as a result, music therapy is effective in reducing nausea and vomiting in these patient groups [37]. In the study of Rhodes et al. which investigated the effects of music therapy and visual imagery on the severity and duration of anxiety, nausea, and vomiting, they found that it significantly reduced the severity of nausea and vomiting and the duration of vomiting also decreased [38]. Ezzone et al. showed less nausea and vomiting in a group of 33 bone marrow transplant patients who received music therapy [39].

2010 yılında Madden ve ark. Müzik ve dansı birleştiren ve kemoterapi gören hastalar için haftada 60 dakika uygulanan bir sanat formu tasarladı [40]. Deney grubundaki hastalar, kontrol grubundaki hastalara göre önemli ölçüde daha az mide bulantısı bildirdiler.

In a meta-analysis study conducted by Zhong and colleagues, seven articles applying music therapy to patients receiving chemotherapy were analyzed. This study determined that music therapy significantly improved symptoms of nausea and vomiting in patients with digestive system cancer during chemotherapy [41]. In the study by Doro et al. it was found that music therapy provided bio-psychosocial well-being by reducing nausea and pain in patients who underwent autologous hematopoietic stem cell transplantation [42]. According to a randomized study conducted by Madson and Silverman in a group of 58 patients who underwent solid organ transplantation, it was found that there was less nausea and vomiting in the music therapy group [43].

A systematic review and meta-analysis were conducted by Wei and colleagues to investigate the relationship between nausea and vomiting and music therapy. Cochrane Central Register of Controlled Trials (CENTRAL), PubMed, EMBASE, Cumulative Index to Nursing and Allied Health Literature (CINAHL), China Biomedical Database (CBM), China National Knowledge Infrastructure (CNKI) and WanFang were searched as databases for this study. A total of 608 studies were examined in these scanned databases. Ten randomized controlled trials met the criteria established for the study. A total of 632 patients were included in the study. The effect of music therapy applied to the patients was analyzed. The study was analyzed by comparing the effect of music therapy with the type of music, duration of listening to music, and frequency of listening to music. The results were that music therapy reduced the expected incidence and severity of nausea and vomiting [44].

In another study by Pozhhan and colleagues, sixty patients were equally randomized into experimental (music therapy group) and control (routine care group) groups. About 148 instrumental, recreational, and religious records were transmitted through headphones connected to an MP3 player. The intervention consisted of five 25-minute sessions supervised by trained nurses to provide the patient's favorite music, volume, and timing regulation. A 0–10 visual analog scale (VAS) and a 4-point Likert scale were used to measure the severity of nausea. Frequencies were also asked and recorded. Study endpoints were determined before, during, and after chemotherapy (8-hours, 16-hours, and 24-hours). The statistical tests performed were found to be statistically significant in favor of the music therapy group in terms of the median of nausea frequency, vomiting frequency, nausea severity, and vomiting severity between the music therapy and control groups. Music therapy reduced the frequency and severity of nausea and vomiting in the intervention group receiving chemotherapy compared to the control group. As a result, the authors suggested that music therapy should be included in the recovery process after chemotherapy in women with breast cancer [45].

Many chronic health problems arise with aging. One of these, high blood pressure, can cause serious complications if not controlled. In addition to pharmacological treatment, non-pharmacological treatment is also widely used in hypertensive patients. The effect of music on the autonomic nervous system is reflected in a positive effect on blood pressure, as discussed before. For this reason, in addition to pharmacological treatment, music therapy can be used by taking advantage of the mechanism of music affecting the neurohormonal and autonomic systems.

Lorber and Divjak investigated the relationships between blood pressure and music therapy. This study was a random controlled study on elderly people in nursing homes. In the study, they aimed to reveal whether listening to music affects blood pressure, heart rate, and anxiety in the elderly. Thirty elderly individuals were randomly included in the experimental group and 30 elderly individuals were in the control group. Music therapy was applied to the experimental group. The experimental group that received music therapy was compared with the control group. As a result of the comparison, there were significant decreases in heart rate, systolic blood pressure, and anxiety in the elderly individuals in the experimental group. Thus, researchers said that as a result of this study, music therapy can be used as an alternative treatment method. Moreover, the fact that it is cheap, does not cause any harm to the person, and is safe are stated as important reasons for the preferability of this method [46].

Cao and Zhang conducted a meta-analysis study to evaluate the effects of adjuvant music therapy in hypertension patients and to shed light on the clinical management of hypertension. A total of 20 randomized controlled studies were included in the study. In these studies, it was determined that music therapy was applied to 1154 patients. The analysis of the study showed that music therapy lowered blood pressure, a vital sign. It was also found to have positive effects on both systolic and diastolic blood pressure. Similarly, music therapy reduced heart rate in this study [47].

Loomba and his colleagues investigated how music therapy affects blood pressure in their study "Effects of music on systolic blood pressure, diastolic blood pressure, and heart rate: a meta-analysis" in 2012. They compared the group that received music therapy and the group that did not. In this comparison, diastolic blood pressure was found to be significantly lower in patients in the music therapy group. Similarly, heart rate decreased in patients who received music therapy compared to patients who did not receive music therapy [48].

Alammar and colleagues wanted to examine the relationship between music therapy and heart rate in adults. For this purpose, they searched six databases (PsycInfo, MEDLINE, PubMed, CINAHL, and Cochrane Library). In this meta-analysis study, there were 194 studies on the subject from six databases. They included 12 studies from these studies. The data of 1.118 adult patients who took part in the studies accepted for the study were included. The patients had different medical diagnoses. At the end of the analysis of the study, it was determined that the heart rate of the patients in the experimental group (who received music therapy) decreased compared to the patients in the control group (who did not receive music therapy) [49].

5. Substance abuse and music therapy

Many studies indicate that one of the unique interventions that can cure drug addicts is music therapy. From past to present, music therapy has been applied variably as primary and secondary health care for people with alcohol, tobacco, and other drug addictions. The data obtained in studies conducted in the field of music therapy suggest that music can play a critical role in multifaceted research. Music can be used to motivate and engage patients with substance addiction, to reveal emotions and positive mood changes, and to reduce stress and anxiety. The purpose of music therapy in substance addiction is to save the person from substance addiction, to encourage the change of existing behaviors that harm the individual or society, and to raise awareness of the basic bio-psycho-social factors that contribute to substance use problems [50]. In a study conducted by W. S. Mathis, he states that music therapy in drug addicts has a potential esthetic input that can prevent the increase of dopamine in the brain regions affected by drug use and reduce substance craving. In an experiment he conducted with Han, Mathis applied music therapy to a group with substance addiction and made another group listen to white noise. They observed that there was a decrease in the desire to use substances in the group that listened to music [51]. In a similar study, three different treatment methods were applied to the group with substance addiction to reduce drug cravings. To one of these groups, only music was administered, to the other, a desire-reducing drug was administered, and to another group, both were administered. As a result, data were obtained that the desire for substances decreased in the group that listened only to music [52].

In a 2008 study, Dingle and colleagues investigated the effect of music therapy on substance abusers' participation in group cognitive behavioral therapy. They sought to answer the question of whether music therapy enables drug addicts to participate in cognitive behavioral therapy groups. This study was conducted in a private hospital. A total of 24 people, 14 women and 10 men, participated in the research. A total of 24 surveys applied to a sample aged between 17 and 52 were analyzed. The aim was to include patients in cognitive behavioral therapy administered in groups at the hospital where the study was conducted. For this purpose, music therapy was applied to substance addicts for 7 weeks. At the end of the sessions, how many substance addicts participated in music therapy and their perceptions were examined. As a result of the review, it was seen that 75% of substance abusers participated in cognitive behavioral therapy for 7 weeks. During the sessions, it was determined that substance addicts participated in the cognitive behavioral therapy group with pleasure and their motivation increased. They received an average score of 4.3 out of 5. About 46% stated that they saw themselves as part of the group thanks to music therapy. About 83% said they would attend other music therapy sessions in the future. They said that in the future, music therapy would improve the sense of belonging to the group. In addition, this study determined that music therapy is effective in all substance use. It was also determined that it could be applied to all age groups and that music therapy increased participation and motivation in all age groups in the cognitive behavioral therapy group [53].

Another study was conducted at a smoking cessation clinic. Of the smokers who applied to the outpatient clinic, 53 were in the study group and 61 were in the control group. Thus, a total of 114 people were included in the study. While art therapy was applied to the study group, health education was given to the control group. Thus, some parameters were examined in two groups. Symptom checklist score, blood lipid level, and high-density lipoprotein cholesterol were evaluated along with smoking duration. In addition, serum total cholesterol amount according to smoking duration and lung function according to smoking duration were also examined.

Low-density lipoprotein cholesterol decreased statistically significantly in both the study group and the control group. Symptom control scores of the study group were compared with the control group. According to this comparison, scores decreased in both groups. However, the scores of the study group were lower than the control group and were found to be statistically significant. High-density lipoprotein cholesterol was examined in the control group and the study group. Although smoking durations were different, it was determined that the high-density lipoprotein cholesterol level in the study group was increased compared to the control group. It was also determined that the smoking rate decreased in the art therapy group. Additionally, lung function tests were compared in both groups in this study, and both smoking cessation and smoking cessation rates decreased after the intervention. Moreover, it was determined that lung capacity improved significantly in the study group [54].

6. Sleep quality and music

In order for music to be perceived, sound waves must first reach the ear. A series of steps then begins that convert these sound waves into electrical signals in the brain. Eventually, the brain interprets these sounds and a triggering effect is created for a series of changes to occur in the organism. One of the daily life activities that music affects the brain is sleep. Music affects regulating cortisol levels and stress hormones in people. This effect increases the comfort of people by ensuring quality sleep. In addition, by triggering the release of dopamine, music makes the person feel good before going to bed and helps manage pain, which is a factor that negatively affects sleep. People react both physically and psychologically to musical activity. These responses to music have significant effects on reducing not only acute pain but also chronic pain. Another effect of music on sleep improvement is related to the autonomic nervous system. Music increases sleep quality and improves sleep by relaxing the autonomic nervous system, which automatically controls many systems such as the nervous system. It is known that listening to music has significant effects on the autonomic nervous system. The autonomic nervous system, which regulates breathing, heart rate, and blood pressure, has a healing effect on these functions with the influence of music.

A study was conducted by Kavurmacı et al. on university students. In this study, pretest and posttest were applied and a control group was used. An answer was sought to the question of whether music therapy affects students' sleep quality. In the study, students who received a total score of 5 or more according to the Pittsburgh Sleep Quality Index (PUQI), who did not have any neurological/psychiatric disorders, who did not have a hearing problem, who did not receive any medical treatment, and who volunteered to participate in the study were included in the study. In this study, after randomization was achieved, students in the experimental group were allowed to listen to music for 1 hour a day *via* a music player. The MPM music player was asked to keep the music volume below 70% from students. The control group was not allowed to listen to music or any other intervention. Both groups continued their normal routines, including sleep. No other intervention was made to either the experimental or control groups regarding sleep habits. Before the intervention, the Pittsburgh Sleep Quality Index was applied to both groups, and baseline values were determined. Then, after the music treatment was given to the experimental group, the Pittsburgh Sleep Quality Index was applied again as a final test. When these measurements were compared, the post-test scores showed that sleep quality was improved in the Experimental Group compared to the Control Group. This value was statistically significant. Music therapy, one of the non-pharmacological treatment approaches for solving sleep problems, has been recommended as a non-pharmacological method that can be used in all areas of health, as a painless, safe, and economical treatment method without any side effects [55].

Another study examining the relationship between music therapy and sleep quality was conducted on elderly people. For this purpose, elderly people living in nursing homes were examined. The method of the study was pretest-posttest single group quasi-experimental. In the first stage, sleep quality was determined with a scale and the baseline value was obtained. Then, the elderly listened to music before going to bed at night, and their sleep quality was measured again as a final test. As a result, it was determined in the study that music therapy applied to the elderly before going to bed improved their sleep quality and they slept more comfortably [56].

7. Conclusion

It is known that the art of music has existed since primitive societies and has an important place in human life. Because people have expressed their joy, sadness, and love through the art of music in every period of their lives. Among the fine arts, music is the area where emotions are best expressed and have the highest social impact. Music, a phenomenon that has been going on since the existence of humanity, is inherently empowering, cathartic, and healing. For this reason, it seems that the use of music as a therapy method dates back to prehistoric times and a wide variety of cultures. Thus, music has played an active role in the belief systems of many civilizations and has been used to treat diseases. Literature review shows that music therapy is widely used in health fields with increasing interest due to its relaxing effect on the symptoms of chronic diseases. As a result of the neurophysiological physiological effects of music therapy in this literature study, it has been determined that music is an important complementary medicine method that reduces heart rate and blood pressure, provides relaxation, changes the patient's perception of pain, diverts attention, reduces nausea due to chemotherapy, and improves the quality of life in patients and healthy individuals. Music therapy, which has the potential to improve symptomatic treatment and quality of life measures, is necessary and important to be used routinely alongside medical treatment, especially in clinical areas.

Author details

Songül Mollaoğlu[1] and Mukadder Mollaoğlu[2]*

1 Faculty of Education, Department of Fine Arts, Sivas Cumhuriyet University, Sivas, Turkey

2 Faculty of Health Sciences, Sivas Cumhuriyet University, Sivas, Turkey

*Address all correspondence to: mukaddermollaoglu@hotmail.com

References

[1] Rio RE, Tenney KS. Music therapy for juvenile off enders in residential treatment. Music Therapy Perspectives. 2002;**20**(1):89-97

[2] Yıldırım M. Music healing: History, development, application in addictions and music therapy applications in Turkey. Turkish Academic Research Review. 2021;**6**(2):477-497

[3] Tièschky T, Mastnak W. ARION psychovocal therapy—Funktionale Gesangspädagogik im psychiatrischen setting. Psychiatrische Praxis. 2016;**43**(8):450-452

[4] Grebene B. Müzikle Tedavi. Ankara: Sanem Matbaası; 1978

[5] Turfan BM. The effect of music applications on patients with multiple sclerosis. In: Afyon Kocatepe University Social Sciences Institute Music Department Master's Thesis. Afyonkarahisar; 2019

[6] Karamızrak N. Ses ve Müziğin Organları İyileştirici Etkisi. Koşuyolu Heart Journal. 2017;**17**(1):54-57

[7] Cleary T. Konfüçyüs Düşüncesinin Temelleri. Çev: Sibel Özbudun: Anahtar Kitaplar, İstanbul; 2000

[8] Rogers P. Music therapy research in Europe: A context for the qualitative/ quantitative debate. British Journal of Music Therapy. 1995;**9**(2):5-12

[9] Pratt RR. Art, dance, and music therapy. Physical Medicine and Rehabilitation Clinics of North America. 2004;**15**:827-841

[10] Boşnak M, Kurt AH, Yaman S. Beynimizin Müzik Fizyolojisi. KSÜ Tıp Fak Dergisi. 2017;**12**(1):35-44

[11] Colwell CM, Pehotsky CA, Gillmeister G, Woorich J. The Orff approach to music therapy. In: Darrow AA, editor. Introduction to approaches in music therapy. 2nd ed. USA: Silver Spring; 2008. pp.11-24

[12] Malchiodi CA. Expressive therapies history, theory, and practice. In: Malchiodi CA, editor. Expressive Therapies. Newyork: Guilford press; 2005. pp. 1-15

[13] Dai WS, Huang ST, Xu N, Chen Q, Cao H. The effect of music therapy on pain, anxiety and depression in patients after coronary artery bypass grafting. Journal of Cardiothoracic Surgery. 2020;**15**(1):81

[14] Updike P. Music therapy results for ICU patients. Dimensions of Critical Care Nursing. 1990;**9**(1):39-45

[15] Thaut MH. The future of music in therapy and medicine. Annals of the New York Academy of Sciences. 2005;**1060**:303-308

[16] Nilsson U. The anxiety- and pain-reducing effects of music interventions: A systematic review. AORN Journal. 2008;**87**(4):780-807

[17] McCaffrey R, Locsin CR. Music listening as a nursing intervention: A symphony of practice. Holistic Nursing Practice. 2002;**16**(3):70-77

[18] Arslan S. Dokunma, Müzik Terapi Ve Aromaterapinin Yoğun Bakım Hastalarının Fizyolojik Durumlarına Etkisi [thesis]. Erzurum: Atatürk Üniversitesi Sağlık Bilimleri Enstitüsü; 2007

[19] Kemper KJ, Danhauer SC. Music as therapy. Southern Medical Journal. 2005;**98**:3

[20] Covington H. Therapeutic music for patients with psychiatric disorders. Holistic Nursing Practice. 2001;**15**:59-69

[21] Raja SN, Carr DB, Cohen M, Finnerup NB, Flor H, Gibson S, et al. The revised international association for the study of pain definition of pain: Concepts, challenges and compromises. Pain. 2020;**161**(9):1976-1982

[22] Altuntaş D, Efe E. Çocuklarda ağrı yönetiminde müzik: Lisansüstü tezler. Ordu Üniversitesi Hemşirelik Çalışmaları Dergisi. 2022;**5**(2):234-242

[23] Stegemann T, Geretsegger M, Phan Quoc E, Riedl H, Smetana M. Music therapy and other musicbased interventions in pediatric health care: An overview. Medicine. 2019;**6**(1):25

[24] Öztürk L, Erseven H, Atik MF. Makamdan Şifaya. 1. Baskı ed. İstanbul: Türkiye İş Bankası Kültür Yayınları; 2009

[25] Karaaslan Ş. Müziğin Ameliyat Sonrası Ağrı Üzerine Etkisi [thesis]. Turkey: İnönü Üniversitesi Sağlık Bilimleri Enstitüsü; 2014

[26] Uyar M, Korhan EA. Yoğun Bakım Hastalarında Müzik Terapinin Ağrı ve Anksiyete Üzerine Etkisi. Derleme. 2011;**23**(4):139-146

[27] Elliott D. The effects of music and muscle relaxation on patient anxiety in a coronary care unit. Heart & Lung. 1994;**23**:27-35

[28] Bolwerk CA. Effects of relaxing music on state anxiety in myocardial infarction patients. Critical Care Nursing Quarterly. 1990;**13**:63-72

[29] Chlan L. Integrating non pharmacological, adjunctive interventions into critical care practice: A means to humanize care? American Journal of Critical Care. 2002;**11**:14-16

[30] O'Sullivan RJ. A musical road to recovery: Music in intensive care. Intensive Care Nursing. 1991;**7**:160-163

[31] Tse YMM, Chan FM, Benzie FFI. The effect of music therapy on postoperative pain, heart rate, systolic blood pressure and analgesic use following Nazal. Surgery. 2005;**19**:3

[32] Allred DK, Byers FJ, Sole Lou M. The effect of music on postoperative pain and anxiety. Pain Management Nursing. 2008;**11**(1):15-25

[33] Takmak Ş, Karaçar Y, Karaçar Hİ, Çelik GK. The effect of nature-based music intervention on adaptation and anxiety levels in patients with COVID-19 placed in the prone position: A randomized controlled trial. Intensive and Critical Care Nursing. 2023;**79**:103496. DOI: 10.1016/j.iccn.2.103496

[34] Wu MH, Chang TC. Evaluation of effect of music on human nervous system by heart rate variability analysis using ECG sensor. Sensors and Materials. 2021, 2021;**33**(2):739-753

[35] Zhao P, Zhao J, Liu H, et al. Effects of long-term exposure to music on behaviour, immunity and performance of piglets. Animal Production Science. 2021;**61**(5):532-539

[36] Chlan L. Effectiveness of a music therapy intervention on relaxation and anxiety for patients receiving ventilatory assistance. Heart and Lung. 1998;**27**(3):169-176

[37] Özdelikara A, Arslan B. Chemotherapy-induced nausea-vomiting to manage the use of complementary and alternative therapy methods. Gümüşhane Üniversitesi Sağlık Bilimleri Dergisi/ Gümüşhane University Journal of Health Sciences. 2017;**6**(4):218-223

[38] Rhodes VA, McDaniel RW. Nausea, vomiting, and retching: Complex problems in palliative care. CA: a Cancer Journal for Clinicians. 2001;**51**(4):232-248

[39] Ezzone S, Baker C, Rosselet R, Terepka E. Music as an adjunct to antiemetic therapy. Oncology Nursing Forum. 1998;**25**:1551-1556

[40] Madden JR, Mowry P, Gao D, Cullen PM, Foreman NK. Creative arts therapy improves quality of life for pediatric brain tumor patients receiving outpatient chemotherapy. Journal of Pediatric Oncology Nursing. 2010;**27**:133-145

[41] Zhong FP, Zhong J, Zhong MY. Effect of music therapy on chemotherapy-induced nausea and vomiting in gastrointestinal cancer: A systematic review and meta-analysis. World Journal of Gastrointestinal Surgery. 2023;**15**(3):471-479

[42] Doro CA, Neto JZ, Kowalski S. Music therapy reduced nauseas and pain of the patients undergoing hematopoietic stem cells transplantation autologous (randomized clinical trial). Research Square. 2020;**23**:1-10. DOI: 10.21203/rs.3.rs-25921/v1

[43] Madson AT, Silverman MJ. The effect of music therapy on relaxation, anxiety, pain perception, and nausea in adult solid organ transplant patients. Journal of Music Therapy. 2010;**47**(3):220-232

[44] Wei T, Tian X, Zhang F, et al. Music interventions for chemotherapy-induced nausea and vomiting: A systematic review and meta-analysis. Support Care Cancer. 2020;**28**:4031-4041

[45] Pozhhan M, Sobhani S, Rasouli AS, Tohidinezhad. The effect of music therapy on chemotherapy-induced nausea and vomiting in women with breast cancer. Indian Journal of Cancer. 2023;**60**(1):87-91

[46] Lorber M, Divjak S. Music therapy as an intervention to reduce blood pressure and anxiety levels in older adults with hypertension: A randomized controlled trial. Research in Gerontological Nursing. 2022;**15**(2):85-92

[47] Cao M, Zhang Z. Adjuvant music therapy for patients with hypertension: A meta-analysis and systematic review. BMC Complementary Medicine and Therapies. 2023;**23**:110

[48] Loomba RS, Arora R, Shah PH, Chandrasekar S, Molnar J. Effects of music on systolic blood pressure, diastolic blood pressure, and heart rate: A meta-analysis. Indian Heart Journal. 2012;**64**(3):309-313. DOI: 10.1016/S0019-4832(12)60094-7

[49] Alammar K, Baker OG, Alotaiba A, Alkhunaizi A. The effect of music therapy on adult patients' heart rate: A meta-analysis. Nurse Media Journal of Nursing. 2022;**12**(3):423-436

[50] Mathis WS, Han X. The acute effect of pleasurable music on craving for alcohol: A pilot crossover study. Journal of Psychiatric Research. 2017;**90**:143-147

[51] Stamou V, Chatzoudi T, Stamou L, Romo L, Graziani P. Musicassisted systematic desensitization for the reduction of craving ın response to drug-conditioned cues: A pilot study. The Arts in Psychotherapy. 2016;**51**:36-45

[52] Yıldırım M. Müzikle Tedavi: Tarihi, Gelişimi, Bağımlılıklarda Uygulanışı Ve Türkiye'deki Müzik Terapi Uygulamaları/music healing: history, development, application in addictions and music therapy applications in Turkey. Turkish Academic Research Review. 2021;**6**(2):477-497

[53] Dingle GA, Gleadhill L, Baker FA. Can music therapy engage patients in group cognitive behaviour therapy for substance abuse treatment? Drug and Alcohol Review. 2008;**27**(2):190-196

[54] Wang F, Chen Y, Li S. The effect of art therapy on reoccurring smoking among youths. American Journal of Translational Research. 2021;**13**(9):10633-10640

[55] Kavurmacı M, Dayapoğlu N, Tan M. Effect of music therapy on sleep quality. Alternative Therapies in Health and Medicine. 2020;**26**(4):22-26

[56] Sarıkaya NA, Oğuz S. Huzurevinde Kalan Yaşlılarda Pasif Müzikoterapinin Uyku Kalitesine Etkisi (effect of passive music therapy on sleep quality in elderly nursing home residents). Psikiyatri Hemşireliği Dergisi-Journal of Psychiatric Nursing. 2016;7(2):55-60

Chapter 6

A Case of Music and Choral Painting in Online Arts Therapies

Irina Katz-Mazilu

Abstract

This chapter presents an art and music online art therapy process with a 19 years old young woman during the lockdown period of the COVID-19 pandemic in 2021. The EFAT-European Federation of Art Therapy implemented social actions offering free online art therapy by some of its members to anyone experiencing difficulties at this time. The author volunteered to offer eight free art therapy sessions in individual settings in 2021 to 10 clients. The chapter describes the therapeutic process that successfully helped the client solve issues resulting from social isolation and other personal and familial aspects. The art therapy process combined art and music in each session with writing, recording, and finally, sharing. The therapeutic methodology, relationship and creativity are presented in their specific and original context. The chapter discusses the advantages and limits of the online methodology and some clinical and ethical questions and refers to other research in the field. While more research is needed on the synergy between different media, this case proves the efficiency of online arts therapies. The originality of this case is to cross music and art – as asked by a very gifted client. The healing power of the therapy is reinforced by crossing the two media and the two partners' creativity: client's and therapist's.

Keywords: music, art, online art therapy, synaesthesia, creativity, therapeutic relationship

1. Introduction

Early 2021, Margherita is a 19 years young woman studying contemporary literature at the university of the city, where she lives with her parents.

The year before, she had a difficult time: "her father left the home to join a new partner, her mother, already fragile, was unhappy, destabilised and clinging on her (daughter...) Margherita has still a good relationship with her father but this event was a shock as she didn't expect it, nobody knew about the parallel life of the father. Moreover, she has had a hard time to be a teenager, to become a woman, she was searching...."

Margherita lives in Italy, the first European country to be strongly impacted by the COVID-19 pandemic. With the first – and strict – lockdown, she finds herself brutally isolated. She keeps living with her mother, studying online, separated from her friends. She gets anxious, depressed, lost.

In these siderating times, between 2020 and 2021, the EFAT-European Federation of Art Therapy – offers support to its members personally and professionally. Working groups, seminars and meetings help keep in touch, belong to a community and maintain professional development. First social action will be implemented between early January and the end of March 2021, offering eight free online art therapy sessions to anyone experiencing psychological difficulties with the pandemic. Each art therapist is free to organise the process (duration and frequency of the eight offered sessions, methods and materials, individual or group workshops, etc.) but has to sign a specific contract established by the EFAT. The characteristics of online art therapy have to be thoroughly explained to clients, and their consentment asked if any further use of their art therapy work is previewed. At the end of the social action, the participating art therapists are asked to deliver a short report. Group supervision is offered by experienced colleagues [1].

I am a volunteer for this action, able to work in French, English and Romanian. Starting from early 2021, I have had the opportunity to offer individual online art therapy to up to 10 clients from several European countries: France, Italy, Slovakia, and Ukraine. But, at this time, online art therapy is a challenge for me as I never practised it before. I feel insecure… Moreover, the lockdown echoes my own locked-in experience in my native country, Ceausescu's Romania, where I lived my young years in an open-sky prison… Through EFAT, I can benefit from four supervision sessions which are very helpful.

2. The arts therapy setting and process

Margherita gets in touch with me in this frame, and we have eight art therapy sessions online in English. She has to find some place in the small apartment where she lives with her mother offering confidentiality and intimacy – sometimes the kitchen, or a glory hole where I can see the vacuum cleaner, etc.

I require Margherita's consentment to take pictures of her work and record the sessions to allow her to view herself in action. She agrees with this method often used in drama therapy and dance therapy. Mirroring oneself is a plus offered in online work.

Margherita is a brilliant and very gifted young woman. Before COVID, she already had experienced painting, music, theatre and dance, and she is writing poems…her wish is to be a multimedia artist exploring the synergy of crossed arts' possibilities. But for now, she feels locked and blocked: is her creativity lost? Behind this anxious self-questioning, I can feel the importance of the family background, her emotional and sexual difficulties, and the struggle to evolve to maturity and adult identity.

Building our therapeutic relationship and acknowledging how to collaborate in online art therapy are the objectives of the first two sessions. They are dense, rich and inspiring. Margherita likes painting with music and asks me if I agree. Yes, of course…she chooses either classical or jazz music, according to her feelings of the day. Soon I suggest painting with her hands, on the floor on big sheets of paper, with liquid materials, gouaches and ink. Her body dances while painting in music.

The third session carried by one of Beethoven's symphonies, Margherita paints with her hands, immersed in painting, her long hair diving into the paper, and finally,

DOI: http://dx.doi.org/10.5772/intechopen.109989

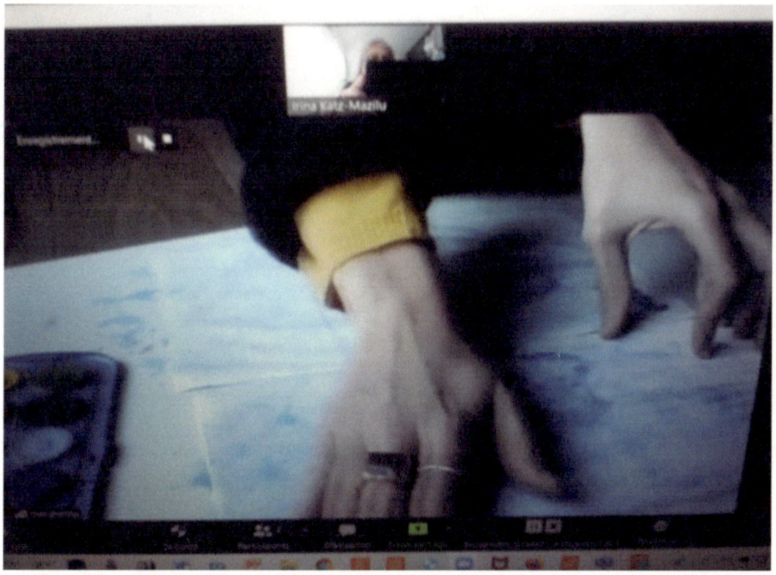

Figure 1.
Painting hands.

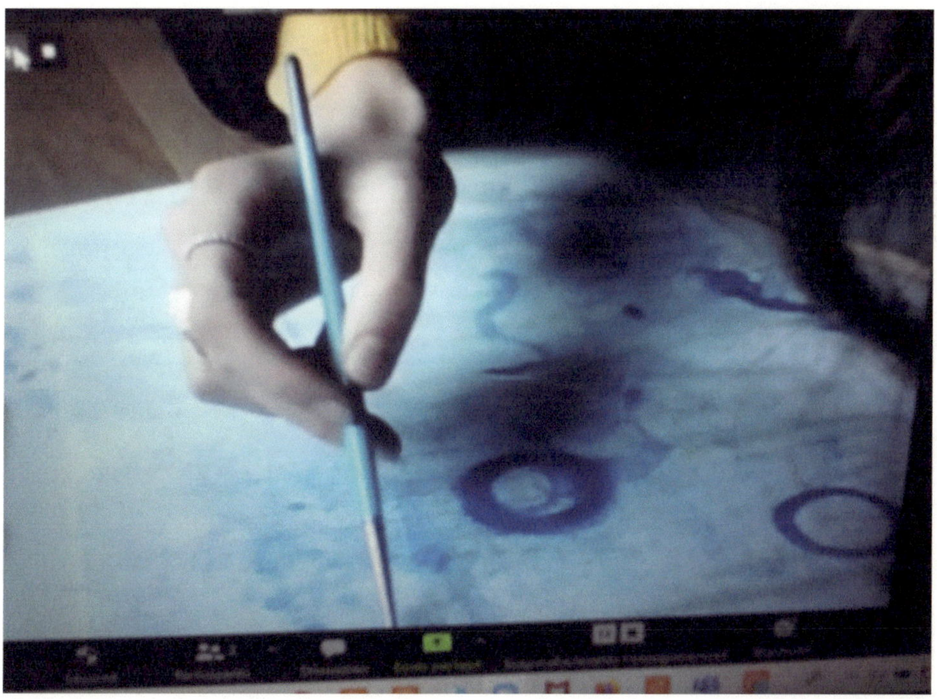

Figure 2.
Hand and brush.

she kisses her painting. In fusion with materials, soul and body in a sensual movement, she *feels,* she is living, she exists... (**Figures 1–4**).

After this third session, she sends me paintings and poems. Her creativity is released (**Figure 5**)

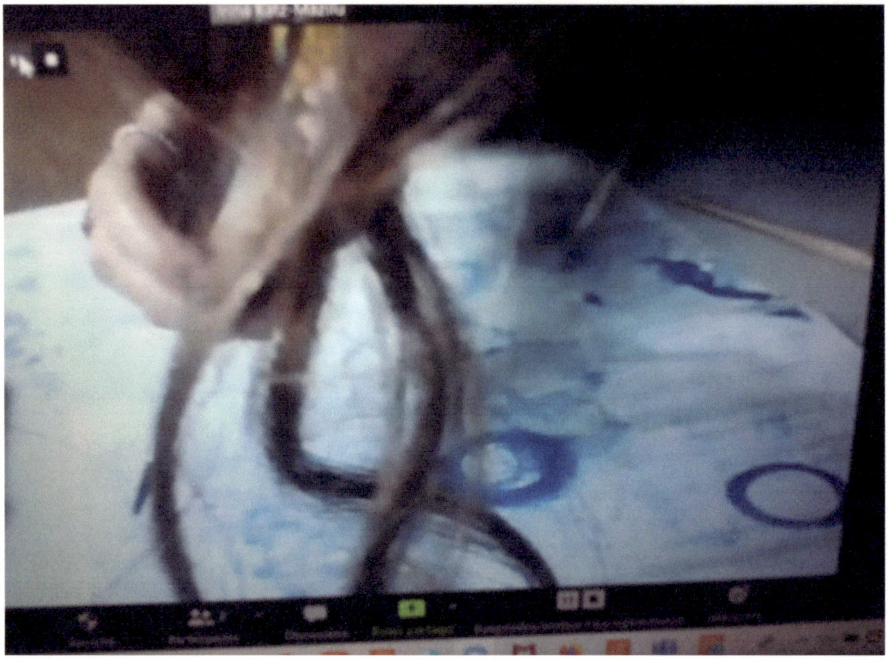

Figure 3.
Painting movement.

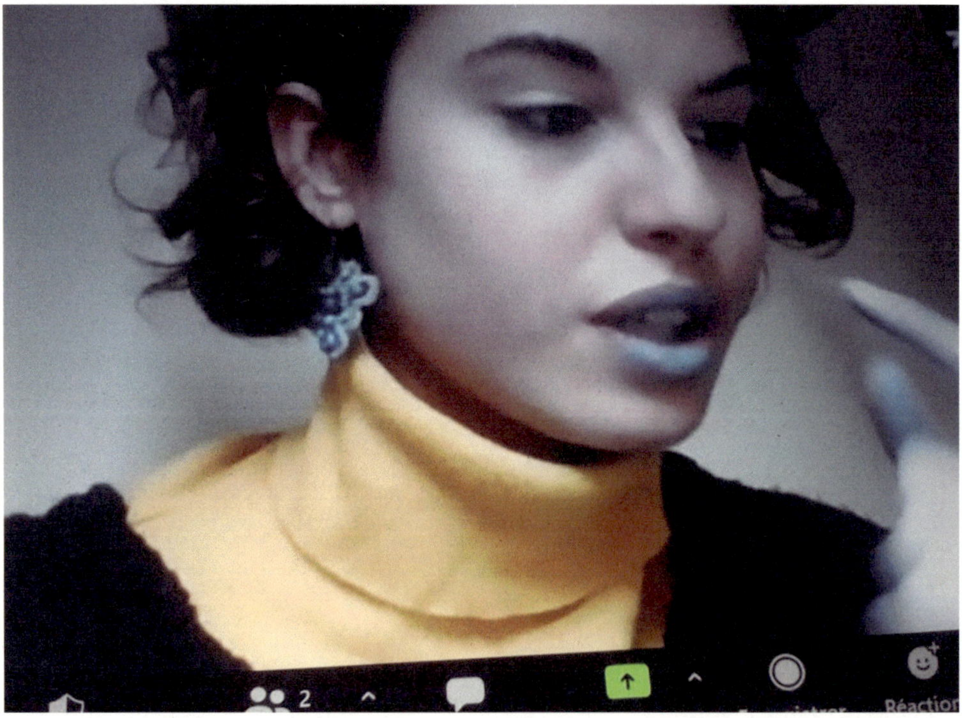

Figure 4.
Margherita with blue lips.

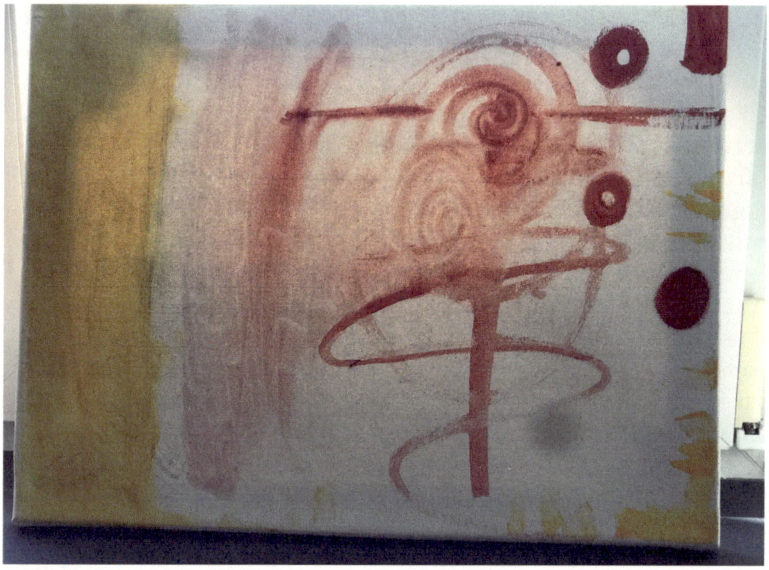

Figure 5.
Dancing figure.

"and these tired shadows

for you today cradle

your hands scratch high on the ground

and shake my lonely steps

there's a world for you

where it's always spring

you living in colours without asking anything in return

these days are sharpened by men,

but I have a place for you in my pockets.

tomorrow morning I'll dress up my twenties

but tonight I am eternal

I don't dwell

because I don't ressemble"

Margherita Fabbri, January 29, 2021, translated from Italian/French by herself.

In the fourth session, Margherita chooses the Heroical Symphony by Beethoven. In her glory room, the vacuum cleaner is like a big musical instrument, and she is her own orchestra director… (**Figures 6–8**).

The fifth session is dedicated to layers painting. Colours and writing follow, recover and transform each other… (**Figures 9** and **10**).

For the sixth session, I propose painting with "real life" raw material: coffee grounds, egg yolk, beetle juice…and mixing the techniques: painting, writing, collage, splitting, holes, etc. This brings her even closer to her body-mind subjective reality. She experiences jubilation with these warming familiar materials, with the freedom to transform them, with the vivacity of her body, with the sensual synergy of the visual, phonic and tactile elements (**Figures 11** and **12**).

She is diving into this original magma. Her defences are lowering; she escapes the omnipresence of intellectual interpretations, esthetically regressing to the age of the free handling of visual and sound stimulations by a toddler[1]. She feels secure in my presence. At the end of each session, we share our impressions and thoughts, coming back to the *here and now.* The regression is contained by the art therapist. Finally, from the original magma, a new structure is coming to life…

She also shows me some of her artwork before the start of art therapy. We discuss the evolutive trends and perspectives. She keeps working on it between our sessions, sending images and poems. A kind of new-born artistic complicity is happening… (**Figures 13–15**).

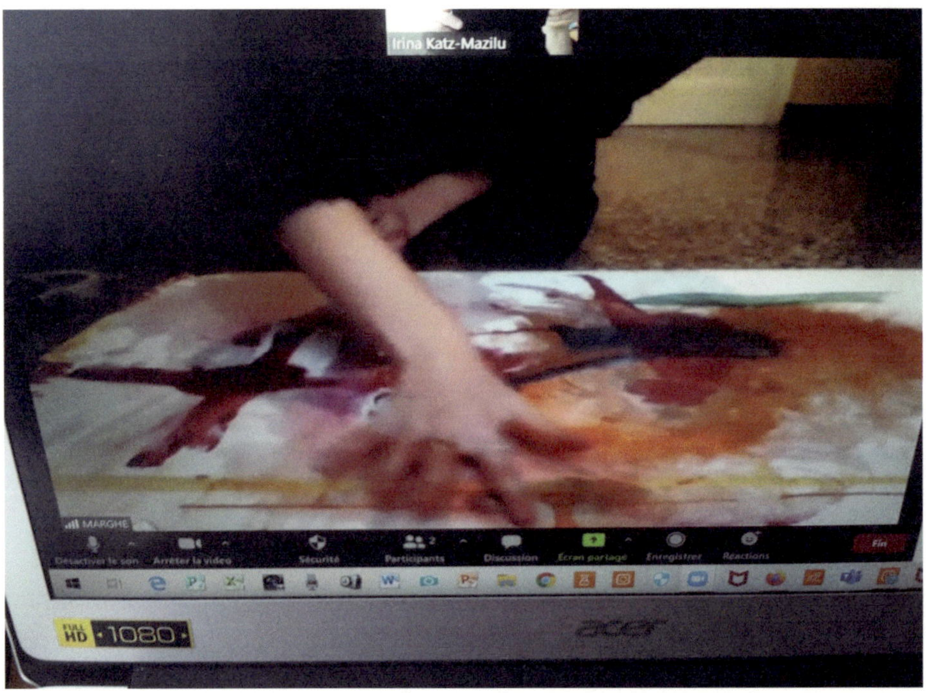

Figure 6.
Finger painting.

[1] The *aesthetic regression* is a concept introduced by Rita Simon as a symetrical concept of regression in psychotherapy [2].

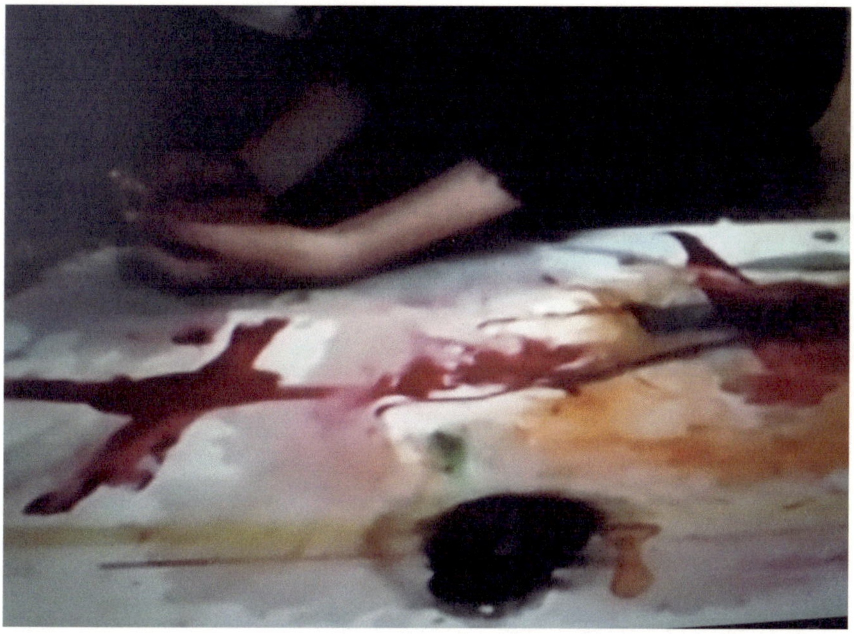

Figure 7.
Painting with the back of the hands.

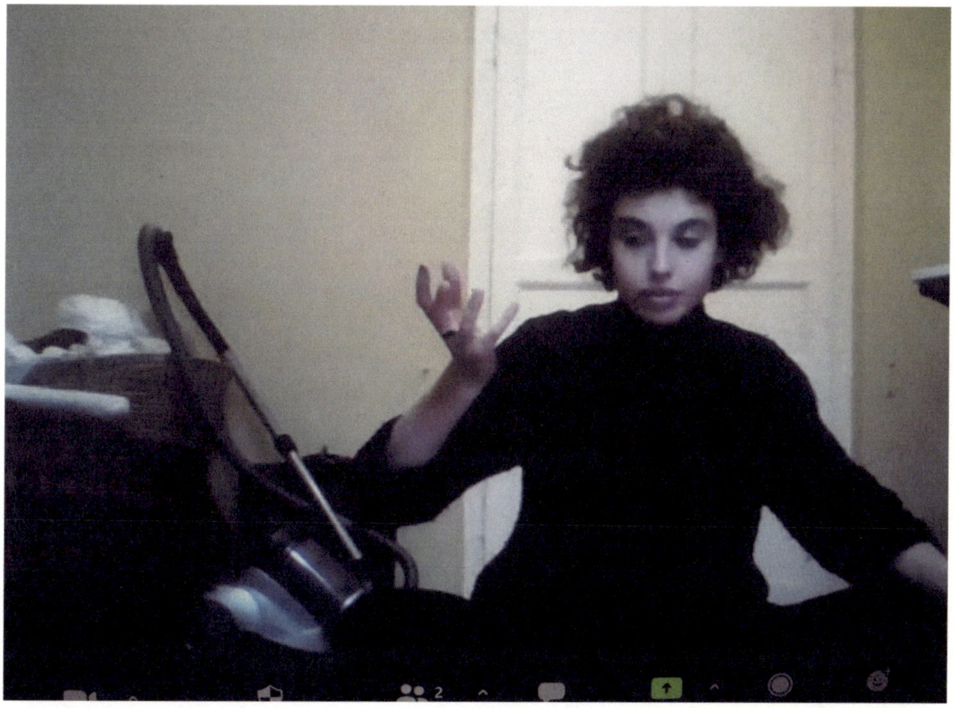

Figure 8.
Margherita like an orchestra director.

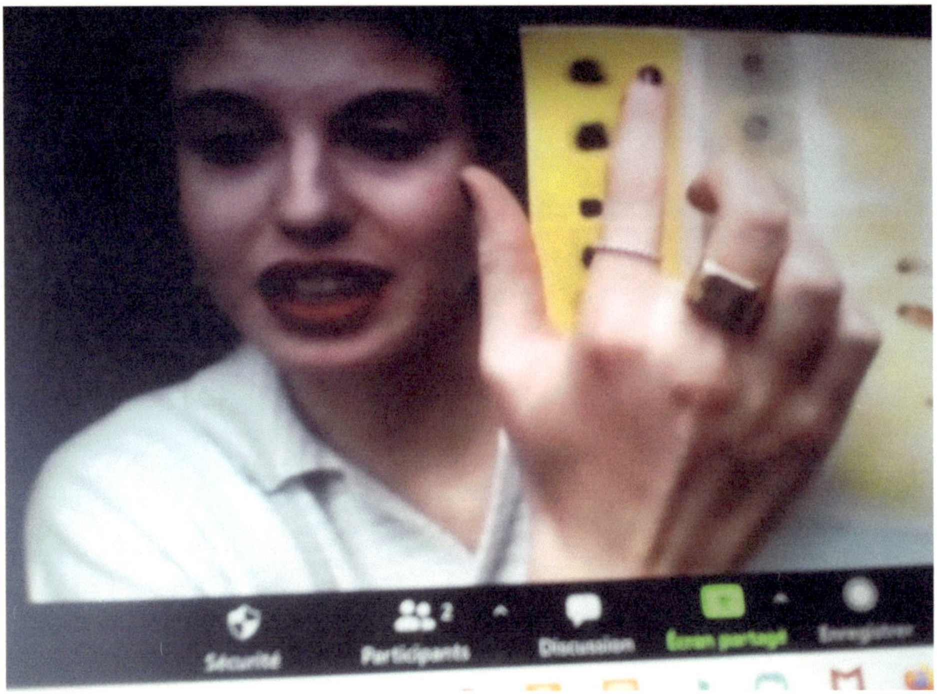

Figure 9.
Margherita showing her painting.

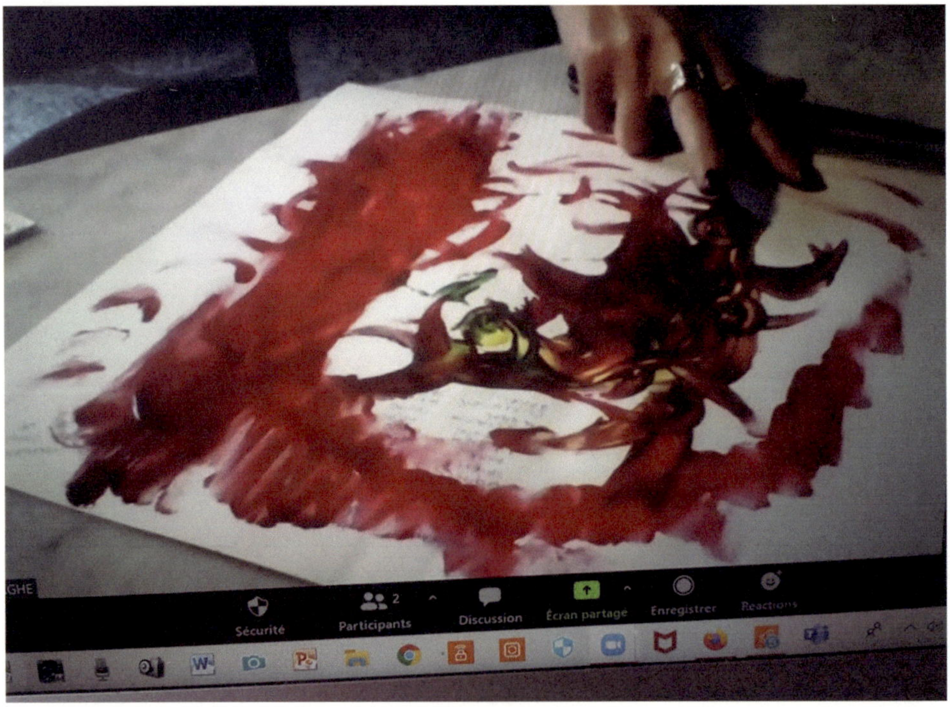

Figure 10.
The red finger paint.

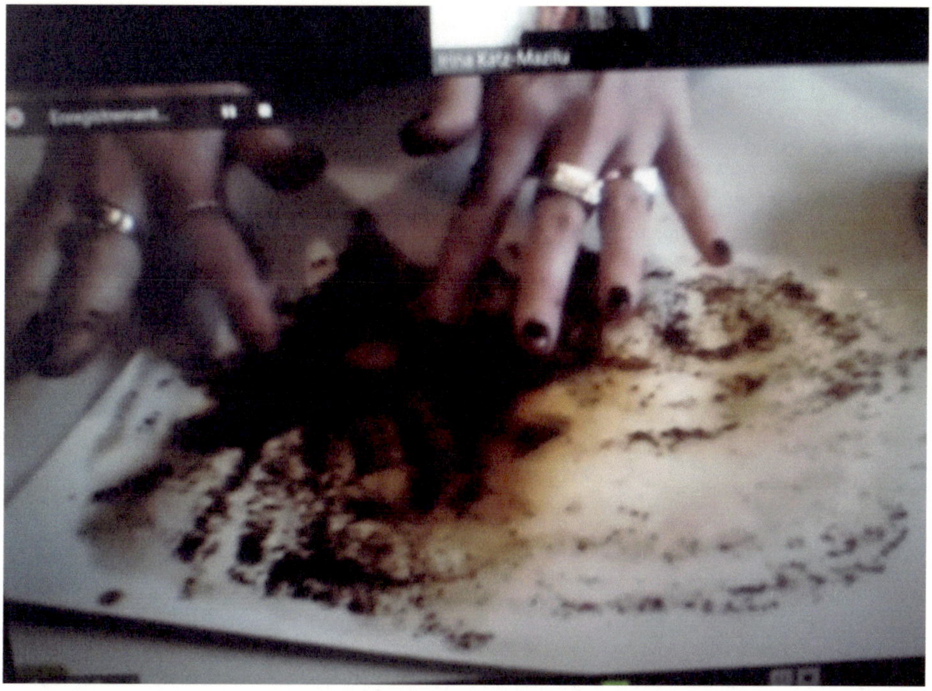

Figure 11.
Painting with coffee.

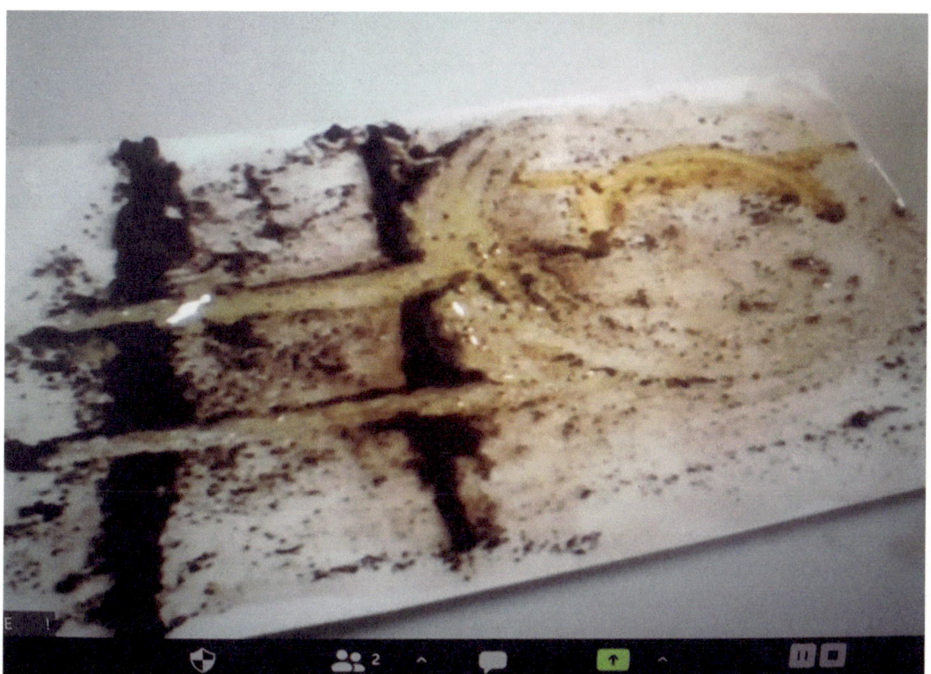

Figure 12.
Painting with eggs.

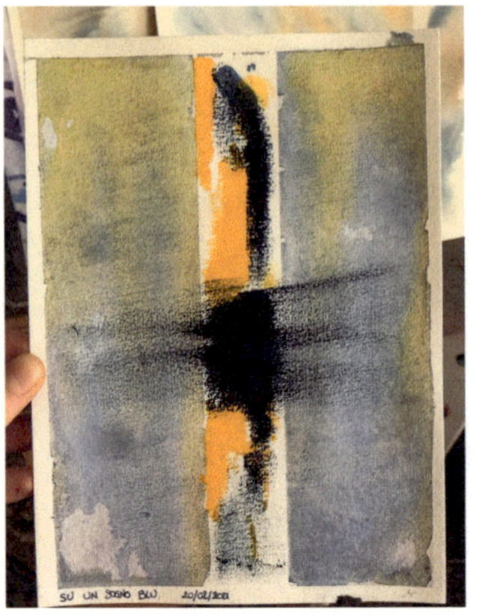

Figure 13.
A silhouette.

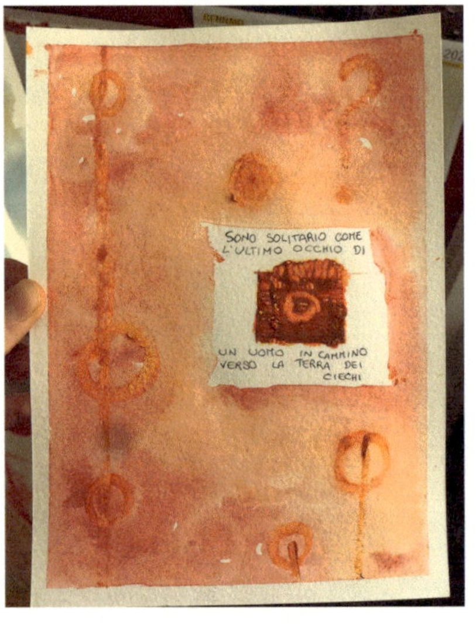

Figure 14.
Painting with a square piece of paper.

Her paintings are now fluid and light. She figures the frame is a protective and mild container.

The seventh session is caressing and tender... (**Figures 16** and **17**).

The eighth and last session is a crowning choral moment of our collaboration. I propose to create simultaneously, each one behind her computer, on the theme of togetherness in spite of the physical distance. We are listening to the same music and painting simultaneously, and the sound is carrying us and bringing us physically and emotionally closer. We feel connected. We show our art and share our feelings. The synergy of image and sound creates a powerful and nourishing stance for both of us. Beyond our therapeutic relationship, we feel belonging to the human community, and we are two human beings, two women, and two artists (**Figure 18**/Irina, **Figure 19**/Margherita).

DOI: http://dx.doi.org/10.5772/intechopen.109989

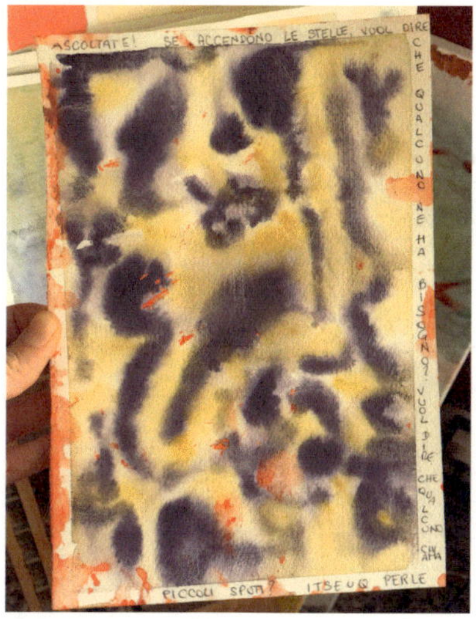
ASCOLTATE! SE ACCENDONO LE STELLE, VUOL DIRE
CHE QUALCUNO NE HA BISOGNO? VUOL DIRE
CHE QUALCUNO CHIAMA
PICCOLI SPUTI? ITSEUQ PERLE

Figure 15.
Yellow painting with black spots.

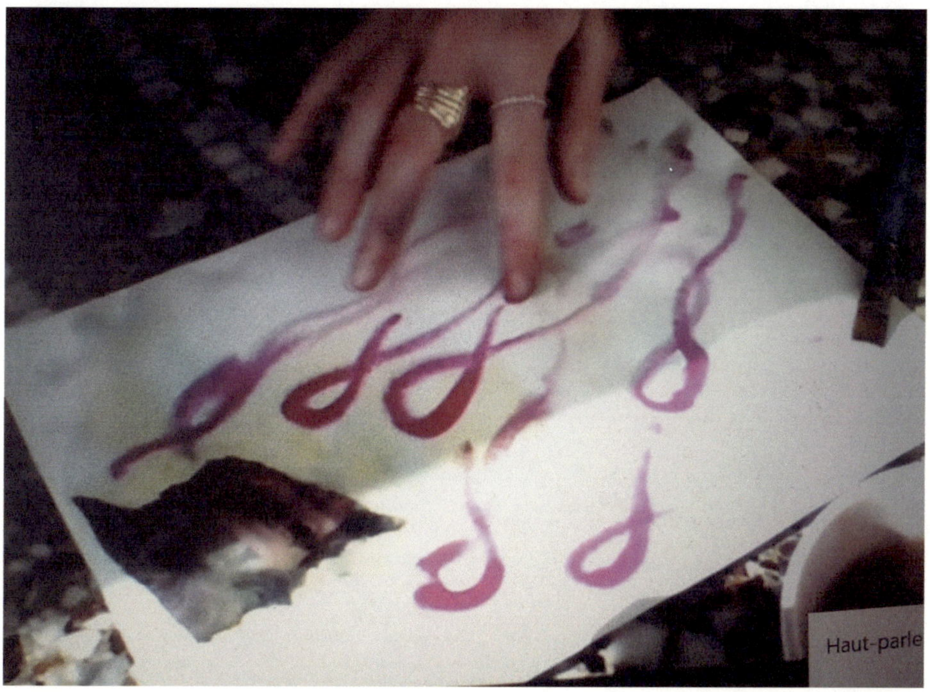
Haut-parle

Figure 16.
Tracing with fingers.

At the very end of our sessions, Margherita showed me a self-portrait she had drawn before her art therapy process. Compared to her actual creative outburst, the change is obvious. This transformation spreads to her relationships with her parents, friends and colleagues. Soon the lockdown will end, and even if the pandemic is not yet over, she feels much stronger to face the challenges to come (**Figures 20** and **21**).

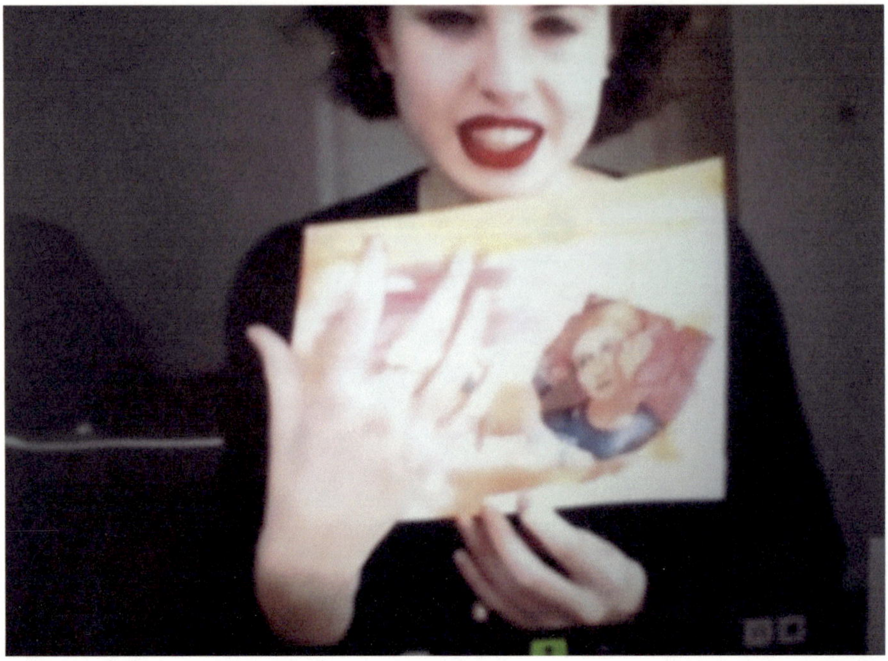

Figure 17.
Smiling Margherita with her painting.

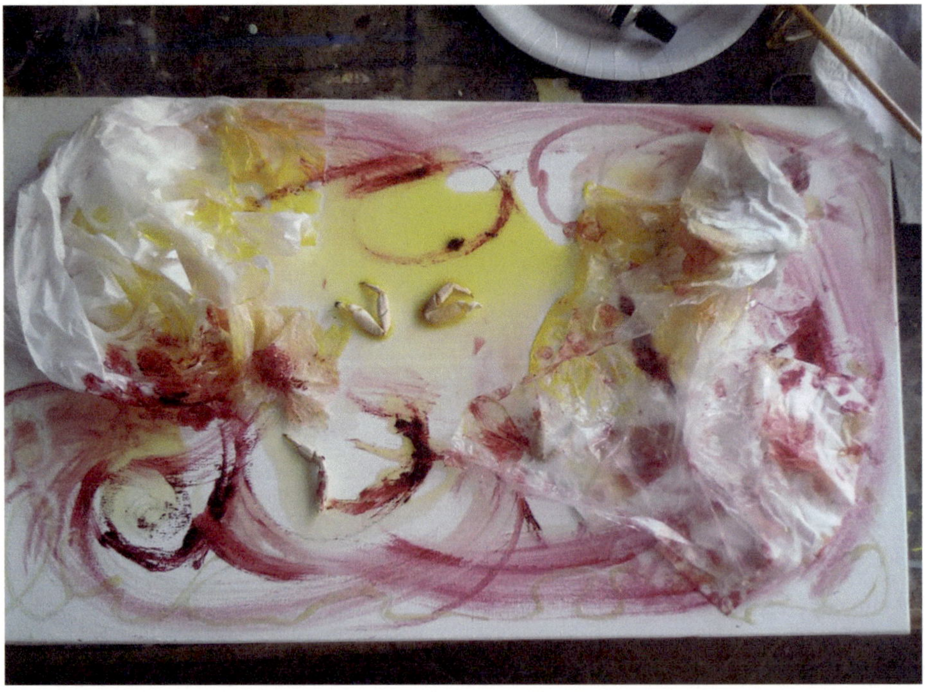

Figure 18.
Simultaneous painting - Irina.

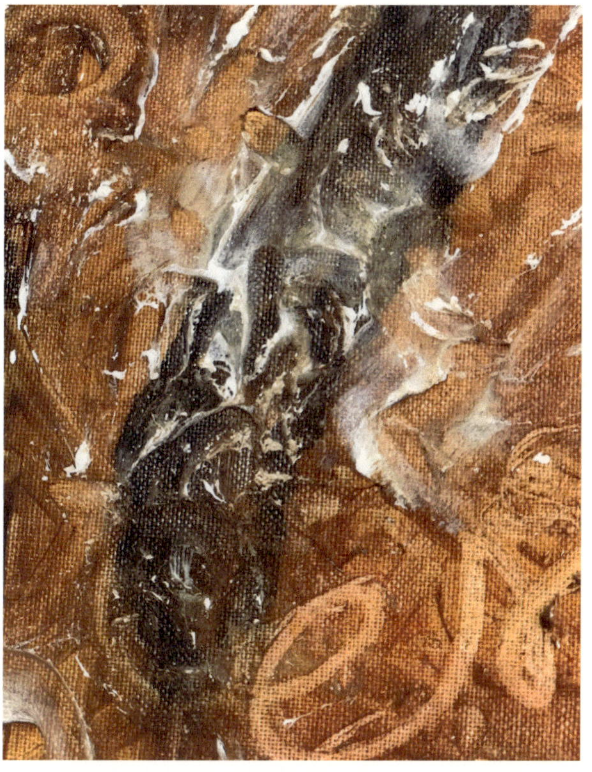

Figure 19.
Simultaneous painting - Margherita.

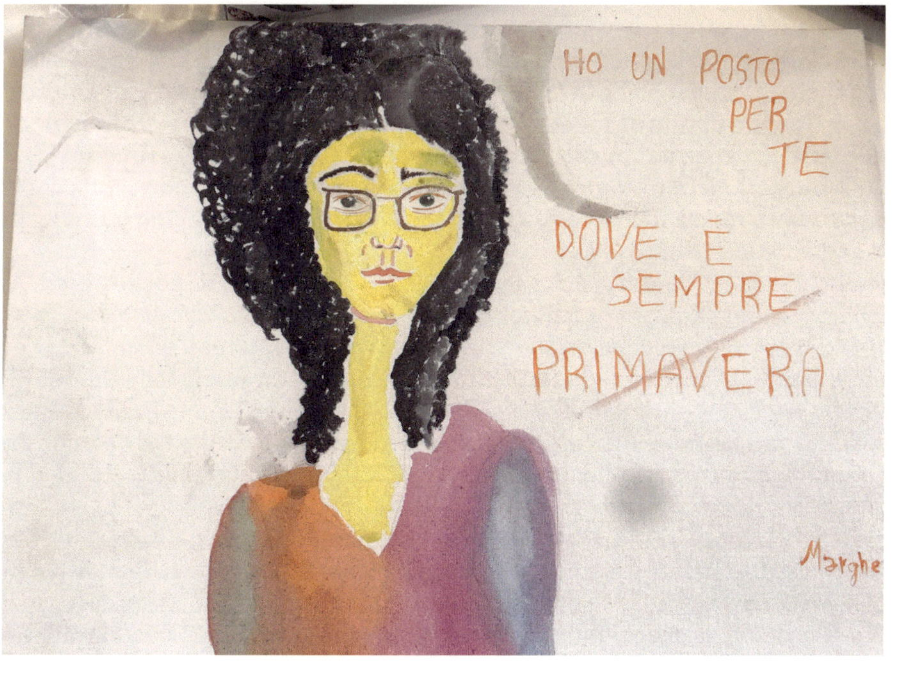

Figure 20.
Self-portrait before the art therapy process.

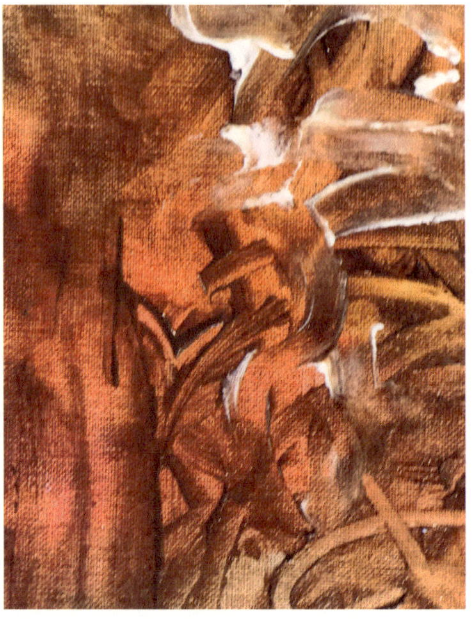

Figure 21.
Fluid painting in brown and white at the end of the art therapy process.

3. Second time

Two years later, Margherita lives in Paris, studying theatre at the Sorbonne University. She starts a new series of art therapy workshops, in my studio, in real life. We were both surprised when we first met: she is much taller than I imagined her online, and my studio is much smaller than she imagined it... This makes us laugh and comment, at which point the virtual reality is biaised...but maybe not more than our subjective perception of the reality? We explore new issues about her evolution, research, travel, expatriation and broadening her life horizon. Each time again, she chooses a musical piece to combine with visual traces. She feels a powerful echoing between the two media in her body and mind. The whole of her being is diving into action and creation (**Figure 22**).

Meanwhile, in 2022, Margherita also published a collection of poems titled "Anime Fradicie" ("Soaking Souls") in Italian.

With respect to the reglementation on the patient's protection, when I decided to write this article, I asked Margherita's informed consent for publishing images of her art therapy work and portraits of herself, as well as for giving some information about her personal and familial difficulties. I also asked her if she wanted to be published anonymously or with her full name. After some reflection, Margherita decided to testify openly and wrote these lines:

"Since when I met Irina and we begun our therapeutical path, I've been feeling the unveiling of something, someone in me, who's not left me since then. A Me in me who's the truest answer to my being. The reason of my consent to using every material without censorship is deeply radicated in this: if there's someone I would want as an expression of me, it is that Me." Margherita Fabbri, January 2023.

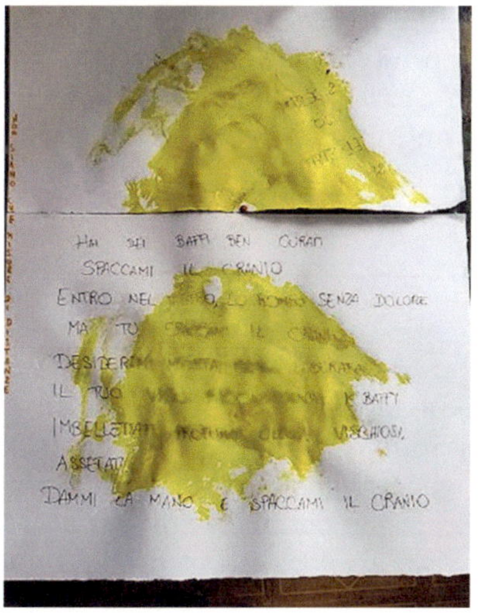

Figure 22.
White and yellow painting with writing.

4. Discussion

Online art therapy at 2000 km distance: did this context facilitate or limit the efficiency of the art therapy? We discussed it without deciding definitively if yes or no, or none of the two...Working with Margherita in this way – and in English – did not damage the quality of our collaboration. It was the only possible strategy at that time of isolation and social distancing – and it proved to be helpful.

One of the advantages of online art therapy is that it lets us free of masks – which obviously is a precious aspect. Also, it allows recording and taking photos/screenshots during the process without disturbing or interfering with the patient's concentration, making it possible to restitute these recorded traces to the patient and discuss each step of the art therapeutic and creative process in detail. Also, for some clients, the physical distance might facilitate contact and relationship.

It would be interesting to check and develop the existing research for a better understanding of the synergy of image and sound in the art therapeutic context by the use of recent possibilities of neuropsychiatry and other medical sciences. The concept of *synaesthesia* helps to understand how the complementarity and the crossed use of our senses can enhance our creativity as well as the healing power of art and art therapy [3].

Nevertheless, if digital technology offers many possibilities, the therapeutic relationship is prevalent in any technical context. Much research has been realised since the COVID-19 pandemic on the pertinence of online tools and methodologies in arts therapies [4].

Several articles have been published between 2020 and 2022 by Emmanuelle Césari and others in *The Canadian Art Therapy Association Online, Magazine* [5–8]. Most interesting is the concept of the "présence modifiée du corps"/"modified body presence" (trad.IKM). The discussion corroborates my own perceptions and analysis of the specific link to the body in virtual settings. We must learn to take advantage of digital techniques and understand their limits.

The specific ethical issues of the confidentiality, privacy, realisation, and the conservation of art therapy products, the sharing with pairs and medical partners, etc., have been the object of a careful elaboration by the EFAT's Ethics Committee and resulted in a Guide for online art therapy destinated to the members of the Federation [1].

5. Conclusion

The use of digital methods in art and music therapy proved to be efficient in the case presented and might be extended to other clinical situations such as loneliness, isolation at home, hospitalisation in a sterile environment, social or school phobia, addiction to virtual games, geographical or social distancing... – when the patients are in a transitory or long-lasting impossibility to join a care centre or a private arts therapist's studio. Music and art are easy to use in a digital context, with simple materials and just a mobile, an Ipad or a computer, in most circumstances. Some existing creative apps might also be helpful for clients who manage digital techniques. Of course, as soon – and if – possible, meeting in real professional life is important because it allows connecting the other's presence by subtle phenomena that virtual techniques and reality cannot offer.

Author details

Irina Katz-Mazilu
Centre Popincourt, Paris, France

*Address all correspondence to: irina.katzmazilu@gmail.com

References

[1] EFAT–European Federation of Art Therapy. Available from: www.arttherapyfederation.eu

[2] Simon R. Symbolic Images in Art as Therapy. New York: Taylor & Francis Ltd.; 1997

[3] Synaesthesia. 2022. Available from: https://www.bbc.com/culture/article/20221102-synaesthesia-the-superpower-behind-great-art

[4] Zubala A, Kenell L, Hackett S. Art therapy in the digital world: An integrative review of current practice and future directions. Frontiers in Psychology. 2021. Available from: https://www.frontiersin.org/articles/10.3389/fpsyg.2021.600070/full

[5] Cesari E, Barberi C. Visio-consultation: art-thérapie en miroir. In: The Canadian Art Therapy Association Online, Magazine. Vol. 5, Issue 2. Envisage, Spring 2022; 2022 [Online]

[6] Cesari E, Clain M. D'écran à écran: un nouveau cadre art-thérapeutique. In: The Canadian Art Therapy Association Online, Magazine. Vol. 5, Issue 1. Envisage, Winter 2022; 2022. [Online]. Available from: https://www.canadianarttherapy.org/envisage/envisage-winter-2022-cesari-clain

[7] Cesari E, Gerard S. Un atelier e-art-thérapeutique avec un processus de faire créatif contre l'anxiété due à la COVID-19. In: The Canadian Art Therapy Association Online, Magazine. Vol. 3, Issue 3. Envisage 3.3 Fall 2020; 2022 [Online]

[8] Cesari E, Gerard S. Un atelier e-art-thérapeutique avec un processus de faire créatif contre l'anxiété due à la COVID-19. In: The Canadian Art Therapy Association Online, Magazine. Vol. 3, Issue 3. Envisage 3.3 Fall 2020; 2020. [Online]. Avaialble from: https://www.canadianarttherapy.org/envisage/envisage-fall2020-cesari-grard

Chapter 7

Relaxing Music in the Dental Waiting Room Has Paradoxical Effects on Dental Anxiety in Patients with High Cognitive and Social Anxiety Sensitivity

Emma E. Truffyn, Colin B. Pridy, Margo C. Watt, Amanda Hill and Sherry H. Stewart

Abstract

We sought to determine the efficacy of a music intervention in decreasing state anxiety and dental-related anxiety among patients awaiting dental clinic services, particularly those with high AS-physical concerns (i.e., fear of adverse physical consequences of arousal sensations). Forty-six dental patients between the ages of 20 and 78 years (61% female) participated in the intervention. While awaiting dental procedures, patients completed the Anxiety Sensitivity Index-3 and were exposed to music selected by experts to be either relaxing (n = 24) or neutral (n = 22). During the exposure period, participants completed the State-Trait Anxiety Inventory-State Form-6, and the Dental Anxiety Scale-4 as outcome variables. Contrary to predictions, participants exposed to relaxing (vs. neutral) music did not report lower levels of dental or state anxiety. Paradoxically, participants in the *relaxing* music condition showed a significant positive correlation between AS-cognitive concerns (e.g., fear of losing control) and AS-social concerns (e.g., fear of public embarrassment) with dental anxiety. Dental clinics should be more intentional in their selection of music in the waiting room, as patients with high AS-cognitive and/or high AS-social concerns may experience a paradoxical increase in dental anxiety from music intended to be relaxing.

Keywords: anxiety, dental anxiety, fears, anxiety sensitivity, music interventions

1. Introduction

Many people fear dental care: the prevalence of clinically significant (i.e., high) dental anxiety is ~15.0–24.3% [1–3]. About 3.7% of the population meets the diagnostic criteria for the most severe form of dental anxiety, namely dental phobia. Avoidance caused by dental anxiety, including phobic-level fears, can lead to dental erosion and decay, periodontal disease, and tooth loss [4]. Poor oral health has been linked to heart and respiratory diseases, diabetes, and oral-related cancers, as well as to major mental disorders such as anxiety, depression, obsessive-compulsive disorder, and eating disorders [4–7]. Indeed, high dental anxiety increases the risk for other phobias, depression, mood disorders, and other psychiatric disorders and symptoms [7].

Unlike other Blood-Injection-Injury (BII) phobias, dental phobia is marked by intense anxiety at the sight and sound of dental equipment and the dental treatment setting as opposed to the sight of blood and/or needles [8, 9]. Individuals with high dental anxiety focus attention on perceived dental threats (e.g., dental pain) and feared dental stimuli (e.g., sight of drill or dentist) [9, 10]. Dental anxiety is related to anxiety sensitivity (AS)—the specific fear of arousal-related sensations due to beliefs that anxiety-related sensations signify harmful consequences [11]. Examples of such beliefs include: a racing heart rate portending a heart attack (AS-physical concerns); dizziness signifying loss of control or "going crazy" (AS-cognitive concerns); and/or trembling eliciting social humiliation (AS-social concerns). AS is linked to, but distinct from, both state (i.e., transitory) and trait anxiety (i.e., dispositional anxiety-proneness) [12]. In a sample of military workers (88% male), AS predicted dental fears but not more general BII fears [13]. Although AS-physical (vs. cognitive or social) concerns have been found to uniquely predict pain-related anxiety [14], no studies have examined relations of AS components to dental anxiety and phobic-level fears, specifically.

Good rapport with patients, allowing them to express their fears, and talking them through procedures can reduce low to moderate dental anxiety [15–19]. High dental anxiety may require more intensive intervention. Cognitive-Behavioral Therapy (CBT) is highly effective [17] but requires specific training and dedicated treatment sessions [18]. More easily administered options, such as music interventions, may be preferable for dental clinics. Focusing on pre-operative music interventions, Thoma et al. [20] found that patients who listened to music (relaxing music) vs. those who did not (i.e., silence) had lower state anxiety prior to dental hygiene treatment. A meta-analysis conducted by van der Weijden et al. [21] examined the effects of playing background music specifically during dental treatment. Results showed that listening to music during dental treatment reduced state anxiety more than treatment-as-usual and that background music provided a small reduction in dental anxiety [19, 21]. Classical music and non-classical relaxing music demonstrated the strongest effects on anxiety. More recently, a study with two meta-analyses of 104 music interventions (coded separately for physiological and psychological stress-related outcomes) revealed significant beneficial effects of music as compared to control groups. Results showed a significant small-to-medium effect of music intervention on physiological outcomes (e.g., blood pressure, heart rate; $d = .380$) and a medium effect on psychological outcomes (e.g., state anxiety, nervousness, feelings of worry; $d = .545$) across various settings (e.g., mental health settings, medical settings) [22]. No significant moderating effects of intervention characteristics were found but a trend for music tempo ($p = .064$) indicated that music with a slow tempo (60–80 bpm) yielded somewhat larger effects than music with a faster or unspecified tempo.

To date, studies have examined the effects of music on state anxiety in the dental context, with few directly examining the effect of music on dental anxiety specifically. Furthermore, AS and its components have not been investigated as individual difference factors that might moderate susceptibility to the anxiolytic (i.e., anxiety-reducing) effects of music. Moreover, studies have been inconsistent in defining type (e.g., relaxing; neutral) and intention (e.g., distraction vs. anxiolysis) of intervention music. Norr [23] found exposure to classical music (control condition) reduced AS-cognitive concerns more than a psychological treatment (i.e., exposure to feared dissociative symptoms; active condition). It was concluded that classical music might be relaxing and, therefore, an effective state anxiety-reducing intervention for those with high AS. Accordingly, the present study explored the efficacy of an in-situ music intervention in reducing general state anxiety and specific dental anxiety among patients awaiting dental procedures. We also explored, for the first time, the potential effects of AS components (physical, cognitive, and social concerns) in moderating the hypothesized anxiety-reducing effects of music. Patients were pseudo-randomly exposed to music intended to be either relaxing or neutral, and completed validated measures of state anxiety and dental anxiety as outcomes, and of AS as a moderator of intervention effects.

Two hypotheses were proffered: (H1) Music condition would impact both state and dental anxiety, such that levels would be lower in participants exposed to relaxing (vs. neutral) music; and (H2) Music condition effects would be moderated by AS-physical concerns, with AS physical concerns positively correlating with state and dental anxiety more strongly in the neutral (vs. relaxing) music condition, due to the dampening effects of the relaxing music on state and dental anxiety, particularly among those with high AS physical concerns.

2. Method

2.1 Participants

Recruitment took place at a dental clinic in northeastern Nova Scotia. Of 57 dental clinic patients invited to participate, eight declined and 49 gave consent (86% recruitment). Three cases were removed due to incomplete answers (>20% missing data) for a final sample of 46 patients [M $(SD)_{age}$ = 47.44 (15.49), range 20–78 years, 2.2% of unknown age; 89.1% White; 30.4% completed university]. Of the total sample of N = 46: 61.9% reported visiting a dentist about every 6 months; 4.8% visited once a year; 19% visited once every 2 years or less frequently; and 14.3% visited once every 5 years or less frequently. No intellectual, physical, or other mental health conditions were screened for given the scope of the study. Twenty-four (52.2%) were exposed to *relaxing* music and twenty-two (47.8%) were exposed to *neutral* music. **Table 1** includes descriptive statistics and Pearson Product Moment correlations. Between-group t-tests and chi-square analyses confirmed the two music conditions did not differ significantly in age, sex, visits to dental clinic (every 6 months vs. less frequently), or levels of the three AS components.

2.2 Measures

2.2.1 Demographic information

Data collected included participant age, sex, ethnicity, education, and frequency of dental clinic visits.

2.2.2 Anxiety Sensitivity Index 3 (ASI-3)

The ASI-3 [24] is an 18-item self-report questionnaire that uses a 5-point Likert scale ranging from 0 ('very little') to 4 ('very much'). It has three subscales: AS-physical concerns (i.e., fear that physical sensations portend adverse physical consequences such

	Music condition						
	Relaxing (n = 24)		Neutral (n = 22)		Test statistics		
	M	SD	M	SD	t	X^2	p
Age	46.25	15.46	48.81	15.79	.55	—	.59
Sex	66.7% female		57.1% female		—	.43	.55
AS-P	4.92	3.80	4.32	4.57	.49	—	.63
AS-C	2.38	2.84	3.55	3.94	−1.16	—	.25
AS-S	6.25	4.63	7.00	4.64	−.55	—	.59
DAS	9.13	3.64	9.27	4.32	−.13	—	.90
STAI-S-6	10.81	3.88	12.29	5.43	−1.07	—	.15

Note. AS-P = Anxiety Sensitivity Index-3 (ASI-3) physical concerns; AS-C = ASI-3 cognitive concerns; AS-S = ASI-3 social concerns; DAS = Dental Anxiety Scale; STAI-S-6 = State-Trait Anxiety Inventory (State Scale only). M = Mean; SD = Standard deviation.

Table 1.
Descriptive statistics and between-group test statistics.

as heart attack or death), AS-cognitive concerns (i.e., fear that cognitive sensations signal dyscontrol), and AS-social concerns (i.e., fear that observable anxiety sensations will have adverse social consequences). Cronbach's alphas in the present study ranged from acceptable to good (.77 for AS-physical and AS-social to 0.81 for global AS).

2.2.3 State-Trait Anxiety Inventory-State Form-6 (STAI-S-6)

The STAI-S-6 [25] is a 6-item self-report measure of state anxiety derived from the 20-item Spielberger State-Trait Anxiety Inventory-State subscale (STAI-S) [25, 26]. It is scored on a 4-point Likert scale ranging from 1 ('not at all') to 4 ('very much'). Total scores can range from 6 to 24; higher scores (>12) indicate greater state anxiety [25]. The STAI-6 has demonstrated good internal consistency (Cronbach's alpha = 0.82 [25]; 0.84 in the current study) and showed concurrent validity with the 20-item full form and 14-item short form of the STAI-S [25].

2.2.4 Dental Anxiety Scale-4 (DAS-4)

The DAS-4 [27] measures anxiety specific to dental health. It is a four-item, self-report questionnaire to which participants respond on a 5-point Likert scale ranging from 1 ('Relaxed') to 5 ('So Anxious'). The sum of the item scores yields a total score that can range from 4 to 20. The DAS-4 has demonstrated good construct and content validity, internal consistency, and test-retest reliability (Cronbach's alpha = 0.82; 0.89 in the current study) [27].

2.3 Procedure

Data collection occurred across five consecutive workdays (see **Figure 1**). Assignment to music condition was achieved by playing 'relaxing' vs. 'neutral' stimuli (detailed in **Table 2**) in the clinic waiting room on alternating days as patients arrived for their scheduled appointments. To best investigate the effects of the music intervention in the real-world context, few controls were implemented. The order of presentation of

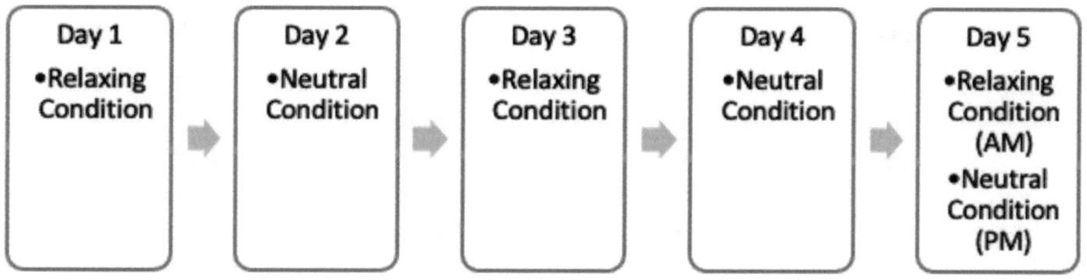

Figure 1.
Music condition design.

the 'relaxing' vs. 'neutral' stimuli conditions were pre-determined; the assignment of the first day as relaxing or neutral was determined arbitrarily. Participants were pseudo-randomly assigned to one of two conditions depending on when their appointment occurred. To match music condition sample sizes as closely as possible, on day 5 the 'relaxing' playlist was administered in the morning and the 'neutral' playlist in the afternoon. Patients were exposed to music stimuli upon arrival for approximately 5 minutes, then were checked in and invited to participate in the study. Willing participants provided informed consent and completed the study measures immediately following exposure to the music stimuli. No incentive was provided for participating. Music stimuli were selected based on a previous study of contrasts in structure between music used for arousal reduction vs. arousal induction [28]. In that study, 160 music selections were analyzed by three expert raters (all musical composers with doctorates) to obtain a single Relaxing/Energizing Index (REI) score for each selection. Each REI score was an average of six equally weighted musical property measurements, each comprised of the mean of three expert ratings. Intra-class correlations (ICCs) were used to assess interrater reliability (IRR) for each musical property measurement. IRR was fair for Rhythmic Definition (ICC = 0.551), good for Metric Accentuation (ICC = 0.719) and Textural Complexity (ICC = 0.670), and excellent for Relaxing vs. Energizing (ICC = 0.875), Intensity (ICC = 0.862), and Tempo (ICC = 0.822) [29]. These REI scores were used to rank the 160 music selections from those predicted to be most arousal reducing (i.e., relaxing) to most arousal inducing (i.e., energizing). For the present study, the 31 lowest-ranked selections (i.e., those with the greatest preponderance of anxiolytic musical structures) comprised the 'relaxing' music playlist (MRelaxing (SD) = 3.32 (0.58)) and the 27 selections closest to the median ranking comprised the 'neutral' music playlist (MNeutral (SD) = 4.94 (0.23); see **Table 2**). The difference in REI scores between the two conditions was statistically significant (t (40.33) = 14.19, p < .001; Cohen's d = .46 (medium effect size)). [Levene's test was significant, F = 17.62, p < .001, so the independent samples t-test was conducted with equal variances not assumed.] Each music condition playlist was loaded onto a Micro SD card and played through a speaker in the dental waiting room. The playlist for each condition was played in a continuous loop and was not restarted prior to each participant. As an awareness check, participants were asked post-treatment whether they had noticed the music; if yes, they were asked to classify the music as relaxing or neutral.

2.4 Data analytic strategy

We (a) tested between-group (relaxing vs. neutral) differences in demographic variables, global AS, and AS dimensions to ensure equivalence between groups; (b) examined H1 through between-group *t*-tests on state anxiety and dental anxiety;

Relaxing music stimuli $N = 31$ songs				Neutral music stimuli $N = 27$ songs			
Song title/ artist	**REI score**	**Song title/ artist**	**REI score**	**Song title/ artist**	**REI score**	**Song title/ artist**	**REI score**
California Stars/Billy Bragg and Wilco	4.11	Adiemus/ Karl Jenkins	3.28	Don't Stop Believin'/ Journey	5.22	Something Good/alt-J	4.94
Crazy Girl/ Eli Young Band	4.00	Canon in D piano music/ Pachelbel	3.28	Dancin' (Krono Remix)/ Aaron Smith	5.22	Lean On (feat. M0 & DJ Snake)/ Major Lazer & DJ Snake	4.89
Matilda/Alt J	3.94	Imagine/ John Lennon	3.22	Blank Space/ Taylor Swift	5.22	Jackie and Wilson/ Hozier	4.83
A Rush of Blood to the Head/ Coldplay	3.94	Lay Me Down/Sam Smith	3.22	Drops of Jupiter/Train	5.17	Chicken Fried/Zac Brown Band	4.83
The A Team/Ed Sheeran	3.89	When you Believe/ Mariah Carey & Whitney Houston	3.11	Every Other Freckle/alt-J	5.17	I'm Comin' Over/Chris Young	4.78
Basket/Dan Mangan	3.89	Between the Bars/Elliott Smith	3.06	Bleeding Out/Imagine Dragons	5.17	Yer Fall/ Hey Rosetta!	4.72
Stairway to Heaven/Led Zeppelin	3.83	Nuvole Bianche/ Ludovico Einaudi	3.00	Sound of your Heart/ Shawn Hook	5.11	Younger - Kygo Remix/ Seinabo Sey	4.67
My Kind of Crazy/ Brantley Gilbert	3.83	Moonlight Sonata/ Beethoven	2.94	Cheerleader/ OMI	5.11	Perfect/ Hedley	4.61
Small Things/Ben Howard	3.83	Love Yourself/ Justin Bieber	2.94	Fitzpleasure/ alt-J	5.11	Dirt Road Diary/ Luke Bryan	4.50
Primavera/ Ludovico Einaudi	3.72	Flume/Bon Iver	2.83	Comfort Zone/ Rebelution	5.11	The Freshman/ The Verve Pipe	4.50
Way it is, Way it could be/The Weather Station	3.72	After the Storm/ Mumford and Sons	2.61	Welcome to New York/ Taylor Swift	5.06	Arrival to Earth/ Steve Jablonsky	4.50

Relaxing music stimuli $N = 31$ **songs**				**Neutral music stimuli** $N = 27$ **songs**			
Song title/ artist	**REI score**	**Song title/ artist**	**REI score**	**Song title/ artist**	**REI score**	**Song title/ artist**	**REI score**
The Girl/ City and Color	3.67	Landslide/ Fleetwood Mac	2.61	Sippin' on Fire/Florida Georgia Line	5.00		
Talk Me Down/ Troye Sivan	3.61	Everything/ Ben Howard	2.50	What do you mean?/Justin Bieber	5.00		
Careless Whisper/ George Michael	3.61	Claire de lune/ Debussy	2.11	Puritan Heart/Matt Duncan	5.00		
Photograph/ Ed Sheeran	3.50	You're The Reason I Come Home/Ron Pope	1.78	Believe/ Mumford and Sons	4.94		
Midnight/ Coldplay	3.39			Crash & Burn/ Thomas Rhett	4.94		

Notes. REI = Relaxing/Energizing Index (REI); scores were a composite of six musical property ratings. Scales and anchors were as follows: Intensity, from 1 ('Very Gentle/Soft') to 7 ('Very Aggressive/Loud'); Metric Accentuation, from 1 ('Very Light') to 7 ('Very Well Marked'); Relaxing vs. Energizing, from 1 ('Very Relaxing') to 7 ('Very Energizing'); Rhythmic Definition, from 1 ('Very Vague') to 7 ('Very Salient/Prominent'); Tempo, from 1 ('Very Slow') to 7 ('Very Fast'); Textural Complexity, from 1 ('Very Simple') to 7 ('Very Complex').

Table 2.
Music stimuli listed by music condition

and (c) examined H2 through one-tailed correlations between AS dimension scores and both dental anxiety and state anxiety in each music condition. Comparisons of correlation magnitude across groups, using *z*-tests, were planned a priori. Given that directional predictions had been made a priori, H2 was evaluated using one-tailed tests. We also explored participants' awareness of the presence of the music and of the music condition to which they had been assigned through between-group chi square tests on the proportions who reported being aware of the music and, of those, the proportions who reported having heard "relaxing" vs. "neutral sounding" music.

3. Results

3.1 Hypothesis testing and correlational analyses

Hypothesis 1 was not supported: no significant between-group (relaxing vs. neutral music) differences in state anxiety or dental anxiety were found. Hypothesis 2 also was not supported: AS-physical concerns were unrelated to state anxiety and dental anxiety in both music conditions. By contrast, dental anxiety was unexpectedly significantly positively correlated with both AS-cognitive and AS-social concerns in the *relaxing* condition but not in the neutral condition (see **Table 3**). Due to the null

	Neutral music condition (n = 22; above diagonal)					
	Age	**AS-P**	**AS-C**	**AS-S**	**DAS**	**STAI-6**
Age	—	$-.40^{*}$	$-.33$	$-.62^{**}$	$-.15$	$-.16$
AS-P	$.58^{**}$	—	$.78^{***}$	$.82^{***}$	.11	.11
AS-C	.00	.29	—	$.74^{***}$	.12	.09
AS-S	$-.33$	.13	$.49^{*}$	—	.25	.18
DAS	$-.13$	$-.01$	$.48^{**}$	$.43^{*}$	—	$.78^{***}$
STAI-S-6	$-.19$	$-.21$	.11	.27	$.80^{***}$	—
	Relaxing music condition (n = 24; below diagonal)					

Note. AS-P = Anxiety Sensitivity Index-3 (ASI-3) physical concerns; AS-C = ASI-3 cognitive concerns; AS-S = ASI-3 social concerns; DAS = Dental Anxiety Scale; STAI-S-6 = State-Trait Anxiety Inventory (State Scale only). $^{*}p < .05$ *(one-tailed).*
$^{**}p < .01$ *(one-tailed).*
$^{***}p < .001$ *(one-tailed).*

Table 3.
Pearson Product Moment correlations, split by music condition (relaxing vs. neutral).

results in the neutral condition, the comparisons of correlation magnitudes across music conditions that had been planned a priori were not undertaken.

3.2 Awareness check

Of participants who acknowledged having noticed the music (21/24 [87.5%] and 18/22 [81.8%] in the relaxing and neutral conditions, respectively), the majority classified the music they heard as "relaxing" vs. "neutral sounding" (15/21 [71.4%] and 13/18 [72.2%] in the relaxing and neutral conditions, respectively). Neither of these between-group differences were statistically significant. This null result for a between-group difference did not change when we compared the proportion of those in each condition who reported having heard music that was "relaxing" vs. "neutral sounding/not noticed" (i.e., using the number in each condition as the denominator: 15/24 (62.5%) vs. 13/22 (59.0%) in the relaxing and neutral conditions, respectively).

4. Discussion

It was expected that patients exposed to music intended to be relaxing (vs. neutral) would report lower state and dental anxiety while awaiting dental treatment. Surprisingly, music condition had no effect on state or dental anxiety, in contrast to previous studies [19, 30]. AS is known to amplify dental anxiety [31]; therefore, it had also been predicted that the magnitude of relations between AS-physical concerns and state/dental anxiety, while awaiting a dental procedure, would be largest in the 'neutral' music condition and dampened (or decoupled) in the 'relaxing' music condition. Instead, AS-*cognitive* and AS-*social* concerns were associated with increased dental anxiety in the *relaxing* rather than in the neutral condition. It appears that for patients with elevated AS-cognitive and AS-social concerns, hearing music judged by experts to be relaxing while awaiting dental treatment may be countertherapeutic.

These unexpected findings may reflect a phenomenon known as "relaxation induced anxiety" in the dental context—a paradoxical effect whereby physiological, behavioral, and cognitive aspects of anxiety are enhanced via relaxation techniques [32]. Our findings suggest that dental anxiety may be exacerbated by listening to ostensibly "relaxing" music while awaiting treatment among patients who fear losing control (high AS-cognitive concerns) or public humiliation (high AS-social concerns) when anxious. The anticipatory nature of fearful thoughts associated with dental anxiety may have contributed to their specific paradoxical increase in dental (vs. general state) anxiety when hearing music intended to be relaxing in the waiting room prior to dental treatment. Furthermore, fears of losing control and being viewed negatively by others may cause increased dental anxiety as these patients begin to relax and "let go" while immersed in relaxing music as they await a feared treatment in a public space. Indeed, high AS has been found to be associated with fear of the loss of vigilance that can occur during states of meditative relaxation [33].

Despite differing arousal-reducing potential between music conditions as previously judged by expert raters [28], most participants in both the 'neutral' and 'relaxing' conditions classified the stimuli they heard as "relaxing". This could reflect differing music perception in expert vs. casual music listeners, a failed manipulation underlying the lack of a differential effect of music condition on state and dental anxiety, or an insufficiently sensitive manipulation check. Importantly, however, the differing correlations with AS dimensions between conditions suggests the two types of music stimuli did indeed produce differential effects that were dependent on levels of two specific AS components. One explanation for this paradoxical finding involves differences between emotion perception and emotion induction in response to music. These are known to be distinct processes and are therefore not always congruent [34, 35]. The majority of participants in each music condition may have classified both 'neutral' and 'relaxing' music stimuli as 'relaxing' based on their *explicit* (or conscious, effortful) perception of musical content, despite differing *implicit* (or automatic) effects between music conditions on the magnitude of the association between AS-cognitive/AS-social concerns and dental anxiety levels.

Music neutral in the tension–relaxation dimension of affect [36] (upon which the Relaxing/Energizing Index (REI) is based [28]) may be needed to maximally benefit dental anxiety reduction in those with high AS cognitive or social concerns. Norr [23] attributed the reduction in fear in his control condition to relaxation (an oblique reference to tension–relaxation) induced by music. Thus, it may be that Norr's classical music playlist (comprised of selections previously found to induce mood of neutral affective *valence*) was also appropriately neutral in the *tension-relaxation* dimension of affect. This may have produced Norr's anxiolytic effects, in line with the results of the neutral (vs. relaxing) condition in the current study. One possible explanation of the anxiolytic effects among high AS cognitive/social concern participants in the neutral vs. relaxing music condition could be distraction—which paves the way for anxiolysis. While relaxing music, like neutral music, would have a distracting effect, relaxing music might also have a counter-therapeutic paradoxical anxiety enhancement effect in those prone to relaxation-induced anxiety, making neutral music a better choice for distraction and hence dental anxiety reduction in these patients in the dental waiting room. Thus, our results highlight two potential processes at play: (1) relaxing music may paradoxically increase dental anxiety in those with high AS social or cognitive concerns; and/or (2) neutral music could be sufficient to distract and hence reduce dental anxiety in patients with high AS social or cognitive concerns.

5. Limitations and future research

Several limitations should be acknowledged. First, caution must be taken in interpreting these results as—apart from ensuring that the two music conditions did not differ significantly on several potentially important confounding variables—few controls were exerted in this study, to ensure the findings were generalizable to the naturalistic dental treatment context. Second, as music stimuli were drawn from a previous study [28] conducted with undergraduate students, the current music selections may have been perceived and responded to differently by the somewhat older participants in the current study. The relaxing and neutral music playlists were based on perceived arousal-reducing and/or arousal-increasing properties as rated by experts. However, these stimuli have yet to be experimentally validated [37] as capable of inducing their hypothesized changes in emotional arousal. It is possible that the neutral and relaxing playlists may not have been sufficiently contrasting to have had the anticipated main effects on dental and state anxiety. Playlists focused on a smaller number of the most arousal-reducing/most 'neutral' selections might have achieved greater contrast. Moreover, it is possible that the exposure duration of approximately 5 minutes was insufficient to induce the expected effects on dental and state anxiety. Indeed, previous studies have used exposure times lasting 15–30 minutes [36, 38]. Finally, it was not possible to determine whether both or neither music condition(s) led to reductions in dental and/or state anxiety. Feasibility constraints inherent to our real-world dental office setting precluded establishment of a pre-musical induction baseline. Future studies incorporating a no-music control group, pre-and post-assessments of state and dental anxiety, and ruling out other potentially confounding variables (e.g., mood disorders, use of other distraction techniques) are warranted.

6. Implications for group therapy

Being more intentional in selecting background music for therapeutic purposes has implications for various settings, including group therapy. Music intended to promote relaxation could induce anxiety in clients inclined to maintain vigilance (like those with high levels of AS cognitive or social concerns). Let's imagine that a well-intentioned facilitator chooses "relaxing" (vs. neutral) music with the intention of alleviating the anxiety commonly experienced by members of a newly formed group. In approaching group therapy, it is not unusual for clients to be somewhat guarded -- wary of group therapy processes, feelings of vulnerability, and of oversharing with unfamiliar facilitator(s) and other group members. Selecting "relaxing" music, however, could have the paradoxical effect of increasing these clients' anxiety and, thereby, impede the development of group cohesiveness. If the group was designed to explore mindfulness, the "relaxing" music could undermine clients' early efforts to become observers of their thoughts and emotions, to let them come and go, to practice self-compassion, etc. all of which require letting one's guard down (i.e., reducing vigilance). On the other hand, "relaxing" music might be more appropriate in later group therapy sessions when the therapeutic alliance among group members has been established and clients' self-perceived need to maintain vigilance has diminished. Early group therapy sessions might be better served by music that is more "neutral" (neither activating nor deactivating) or by no music at all.

7. Conclusion

Many dental clinics use music to relax patients and/or provide distraction from fear-inducing sounds (e.g., dental drills). Results of the present study, however, belie the assumption that the presence of music rated as relaxing by experts will effectively relax patients while awaiting dental treatment. Up to 20% of dental patients are at heightened risk of treatment avoidance due to high AS [22]. The current results suggest that a more intentional (vs. random, i.e., relying on radio or internet playlists) approach to the selection of "neutral" music (i.e., neither extremely arousal-inducing nor arousal-reducing) may best achieve the goals of reduced dental anxiety and preventing future avoidance of dental care among high AS patients.

Acknowledgements

The authors would like to acknowledge the contributions of dental hygienist Michelle Duchovni, clinical staff, and our dental patient participants. Dr. Brad Stark, Dr. Fiona Ryan, and Dr. Colin Pridy completed music analyses [28], with additional assistance from Dr. Christopher Lively. Financial support was provided to the first author by the Nova Scotia Health Research Foundation. The last author is supported through a Tier 1 Canada Research Chair in Addictions and Mental Health.

Conflict of interest

The authors declare no conflict of interest.

Author details

Emma E. Truffyn[1], Colin B. Pridy[2], Margo C. Watt[3], Amanda Hill[4] and Sherry H. Stewart[2*]

1 University of Guelph, Guelph, Ontario, Canada

2 Dalhousie University, Halifax, NS, Canada

3 Saint Francis Xavier University, Antigonish, NS, Canada

4 River Hill Dental, New Glasgow, NS, Canada

*Address all correspondence to: sherry.h.stewart@gmail.com

References

[1] Campbell J. Dental Anxiety - What Are We Missing [Internet]. 2015. Available from: https://www.oralhealthgroup.com/features/dental-anxiety-what-are-we-missing/ [Accessed: September 13, 2023]

[2] Armfield JM, Heaton LJ. Management of fear and anxiety in the dental clinic: A review. Australian Dental Journal. 2013;**58**(4):390-407. DOI: 10.1111/adj.12119

[3] Oosterink FM, De Jongh A, Hoogstraten J. Prevalence of dental fear and phobia relative to other fear and phobia subtypes. European Journal of Oral Sciences. 2009;**117**(2):135-143. DOI: 10.1111/j.1600-0722.2008.00602.x

[4] Sheiham A, Williams DM, Weyant RJ, Glick M, Naidoo S, Eisele JL, et al. Billions with oral disease: A global health crisis-a call to action. Journal of the American Dental Association (1939). 2015;**146**(12):861-864. DOI: 10.1016/j.adaj.2015.09.019

[5] Chalmers NI, Wislar JS, Boynes SG, Doherty M, Novy BB. Improving health in the United States: Oral health is key to overall health. Journal of the American Dental Association (1939). 2017;**148**(7):477-480. DOI: 10.1016/j.adaj.2017.04.031

[6] Kisely S. No mental health without oral health. Canadian Journal of Psychiatry. 2016;**61**(5):277-282. DOI: 10.1177/0706743716632523

[7] Halonen H, Nissinen J, Lehtiniemi H, Salo T, Riipinen P, Miettunen J. The association between dental anxiety and psychiatric disorders and symptoms: A systematic review. Clinical Practice and Epidemiology in Mental Health. 2018;**14**:207-222. DOI: 10.2174/1745017901814010207

[8] Diagnostic and Statistical Manual of Mental Disorders. 5th ed. Washington, D.C: American Psychiatric Association; 2013. DOI: 10.1176/appi.books.9780890425596

[9] Scharmuller W, Ubel S, Leutgeb V, Schoengassner F, Wabnegger A, Schienle A. Do not think about pain: Neural correlates of attention guiding during visual symptom provocation in dental phobia: An fMRI study. Brain Research. 2014;**1566**:69-76. DOI: 10.1016/j.brainres.2014.04.017

[10] Bodner E, Iancu I. Recalling the threat: Dental anxiety in patients waiting for dental surgery. The Israel Journal of Psychiatry and Related Sciences. 2013;**50**(1):61-66

[11] Reiss S, McNally RJ. The expectancy model of fear. In: Reiss S, Bootzin RR, editors. Theoretical Issues in Behavior Therapy. 1985. pp. 107-121

[12] Hovenkamp-Hermelink JHM, van der Veen DC, Oude Voshaar RC, Batelaan NM, Penninx BWJH, Jeronimus BF, et al. Anxiety sensitivity, its stability and longitudinal association with severity of anxiety symptoms. Scientific Reports. 2019;**9**(1):4314. DOI: 10.1038/s41598-019-39931-7

[13] Kılıç C, Ak S, Ak HB. Anxiety sensitivity: Another reason to separate dental fears from blood-injury fears? Journal of Anxiety Disorders. 2014;**28**(2):280-282. DOI: 10.1016/j.janxdis.2014.01.001

[14] Olthuis JV, Watt MC, Mackinnon SP, Potter SM, Stewart SH. The nature

of the association between anxiety sensitivity and pain-related anxiety: Evidence from correlational and intervention studies. Cognitive Behaviour Therapy. 2015;**44**(5):423-440. DOI: 10.1080/16506073.2015.1048823

[15] Appukuttan DP. Strategies to manage patients with dental anxiety and dental phobia: Literature review. Clinical, Cosmetic and Investigational Dentistry. 2016;**8**:35-50. DOI: 10.2147/CCIDE.S63626

[16] Botto RW, Donate-Bartfield E, Nihill P. Chairside techniques for reducing dental fear. In: Mostofsky DI, Forgione AG, Giddon DB, editors. Behavioral Dentistry. Oxford: Blackwell; 2006. pp. 115-125

[17] Gordon D, Heimberg RG, Tellez M, Ismail AI. A critical review of approaches to the treatment of dental anxiety in adults. Journal of Anxiety Disorders. 2013;**27**(4):365-378. DOI: 10.1016/j.janxdis.2013.04.002

[18] Twiss E, Seaver J, McCaffrey R. The effect of music listening on older adults undergoing cardiovascular surgery. Nursing in Critical Care. 2006;**11**(5):224-231. DOI: 10.1111/j.1478-5153.2006.00174.x

[19] Lahmann C, Schoen R, Henningsen P, Ronel J, Muehlbacher M, Loew T, et al. Brief relaxation versus music distraction in the treatment of dental anxiety: A randomized controlled clinical trial. Journal of the American Dental Association. 2008;**139**(3):317-324. DOI: 10.14219/jada.archive.2008.0161

[20] Thoma MV, Zemp M, Kreienbühl L, Hofer D, Schmidlin PR, Attin T, et al. Effects of music listening on pre-treatment anxiety and stress levels in a dental hygiene recall population. International Journal of Behavioral Medicine. 2015;**22**(4):498-505. DOI: 10.1007/s12529-014-9439-x

[21] van der Weijden FN, Hussain AM, Tang L, Slot DE. The effect of playing background music during dental treatment on dental anxiety and physiological parameters: A systematic review and meta-analysis. Psychology of Music. 2022;**50**(2):365-388. DOI: 10.1177/0305735621998439

[22] De Witte M, Spruit A, van Hooren S, Moonen X, Stams GJ. Effects of music interventions on stress-related outcomes: A systematic review and two meta-analyses. Health Psychology Review. 2020;**14**(2):294-324. DOI: 10.1080/17437199.2019.1627897

[23] Norr AM. Amelioration of anxiety sensitivity cognitive concerns: Exposure to dissociative symptoms [thesis]. Tallahassee: Florida State University; 2016

[24] Taylor S, Zvolensky MJ, Cox BJ, Deacon B, Heimberg RG, Ledley DR, et al. Robust dimensions of anxiety sensitivity: Development and initial validation of the Anxiety Sensitivity Index-3. Psychological Assessment. 2007;**19**(2):176-188. DOI: 10.1037/1040-3590.19.2.176

[25] Marteau TM, Bekker H. The development of a six-item short-form of the state scale of the Spielberger State-Trait Anxiety Inventory (STAI). The British Journal of Clinical Psychology. 1992;**31**(3):301-306. DOI: 10.1111/j.2044-8260.1992.tb00997.x

[26] Spielberger CD. Spielberger State-Trait Anxiety Inventory. Corsini Encyclopedia of Psychology. Hoboken: John Wiley & Sons, Inc.; 2010. DOI: 10.1002/9780470479216.corpsy0943

[27] Corah NL. Development of a dental anxiety scale. Journal of

Dental Research. 1969;**48**(4):596. DOI: 10.1177/00220345690480041801

[28] Pridy CB, Watt MC. Structural differences in music endorsed for anxiety sensitivity-related emotion regulation during everyday scenarios. In: 78th Annual CPA National Convention; 7-10 June 2017; Toronto, Canada

[29] Hallgren KA. Computing inter-rater reliability for observational data: An overview and tutorial. Tutorials in Quantitative Methods for Psychology. 2012;**8**:23-34. DOI: 10.20982/tqmp.08.1.p023

[30] Yamashita K, Kibe T, Ohno S, Kohjitani A, Sugimura M. The effects of music listening during extraction of the impacted mandibular third molar on the autonomic nervous system and psychological state. Journal of Oral and Maxillofacial Surgery. 2019;**77**(6):1153.e1-1153.e8. DOI: 10.1016/j.joms.2019.02.028

[31] Horenstein A, Potter CM, Heimberg RG. How does anxiety sensitivity increase risk of chronic medical conditions? Clinical Psychology: Science and Practice. 2018;**25**(3):e12248. DOI: 10.1111/cpsp.12248

[32] Adler CM, Craske MG, Barlow DH. Relaxation-induced panic (RIP): When resting isn't peaceful. Integrative Psychiatry. 1987;**5**(2):94-100

[33] Tsao JCI, Craske MG. Fear of loss of vigilance: Development and preliminary validation of a self-report instrument. Depression and Anxiety. 2003;**18**(4):177-186. DOI: 10.1002/da.10074

[34] Juslin PN, Sakka L. Neural correlates of music and emotion. In: Thaut MH, Hodges DA, editors. The Oxford Handbook of Music and the Brain. Oxford: Oxford University Press; 2019. pp. 284-332

[35] Bradt J, Dileo C, Shim M. Music interventions for preoperative anxiety. Cochrane Database of Systematic Reviews. 2013;**6**:CD006908. DOI: 10.1002/14651858.CD006908.pub2

[36] Schimmack U, Grob A. Dimensional models of core affect: A quantitative comparison by means of structural equation modeling. European Journal of Personality. 2000;**14**(4):325-345. DOI: 10.1002/1099-0984(200007/08)14:4<325::AID-PER380>3.0.CO;2-I

[37] Västfjäll D. Emotion induction through music: A review of the musical mood induction procedure. Musicae Scientiae, Spec Issue, 2001-2002. 2002;**5**(1_suppl):179-212. DOI: 10.1177/10298649020050S107

[38] Lehrner J, Marwinski G, Lehr S, Johren P, Deecke L. Ambient odors of orange and lavender reduce anxiety and improve mood in a dental office. Physiology & Behavior. 2005;**86**(1-2):92-95. DOI: 10.1016/j.physbeh.2005.06.031

Chapter 8

The Use of Music and Brain Stimulation in Clinical Settings: Frontiers and Novel Approaches for Rehabilitation in Pathological Aging

Mariangela Lippolis, Francesco Carlomagno, Fulvia Francesca Campo and Elvira Brattico

Abstract

Aging is a phase of life characterized by the increasing risk of occurring neurodegenerative pathologies, as well as stroke and physical decline. Patients in such clinical conditions are known to benefit from programs able to promote the improvement of associated cognitive, functional, and behavioral disorders. In recent times, growing empirical evidence showed the efficacy of active and passive music-based interventions to be the highest when used for healing these diseases. Additionally, very latest research found the combination of electrical neurostimulation with music to have potential utility for clinical older adult populations, as it may amplify the impulse to neuroplasticity and, by consequence, the rehabilitation gains. Reiterating of active music making induces changes in multiple brain regions bringing to the enhancement of cognitive and sensorimotor skills, while merely listening to pleasurable music stimulates dopaminergic regions of the brain improving cognition, motivation, and mood in a variety of neurological diseases. The versatility of music-based interventions in combination with new technologies allows an effective application of innovative therapeutic techniques. Moreover, their easy implementation in healthcare settings and their positive effects on both recovery and patients' quality of life makes the integration of music-based interventions with conventional rehabilitation approaches highly desirable.

Keywords: aging, music-based interventions, neuroplasticity, rehabilitation, brain stimulation

1. Introduction

Over the years, thanks to the scientific research progress applied to medicine, lifestyle, and awareness of risk factors, our society has witnessed an exponential increment in the elderly population (age > 65 years), and the maximum duration of life has undergone a significant increase compared to the past. As a consequence, the number of people over the age of 60 years has risen up to 1 billion in 2019 and will more than double by 2050 [1]. Reasonably, this poses crucial issues for economies and welfare systems. Moreover, efforts to promote health in the elderly population lag far behind the current situation, making the decline in quality of life (QOL) in older people a major social problem. In particular, physical aging and its consequences are harmful to psychological health and cause the onset of negative emotional states and disabling problems, thus posing a threat to older people's autonomy in everyday life and mental health. Due to these emergencies and to the lack of effective treatments for neurodegenerative diseases, the scientific community has been stimulated to explore the validity of a wide range of rehabilitative and psychosocial interventions defined as nonpharmacological treatments [2]. In addition, while brain reorganization capacity was previously thought to be limited to early childhood, the discovery that neuroplasticity continues with age has led to the development of tools and techniques to promote it even during aging in order to cope with functional and cognitive decline and strengthen already existing skills [3].

Among the interventions able to benefit older people, music started to be widely explored in recent years in order to be included in programs for the promotion of psycho-physical health and to aid the rehabilitation of specific pathologies. By consequence, the beneficial effect of music-based training and treatments has become an object of study in relation to a variety of clinical populations together with healthy individuals [4, 5]. The interest toward music as a means to support the rehabilitation process and its use in clinical settings find reason in the intrinsic power of music to generate plastic changes in the brain and its possibility to act upon the cellular level in both humans and animals. In fact, similarly to sport, music training and listening are able to activate the body and the reward system in the brain [6]. Mostly, the reiteration of these activities triggers the neurotrophic factors (i.e., biomolecules that help both young and adult neurons to grow, survive, and differentiate) including the brain-derived neurotrophic factor (BDNF), a pivotal molecule involved in neuronal plastic changes related to learning and memory [7]. Taking into account the results already obtained from animal studies [8, 9], music could be contemplated as a promising option for improving human brain functioning through fostering the production of the BDNF, which levels are important to be adequate in both normal and pathological aging, and therefore stimulating the neuroplasticity process [10].

According to the recent findings from network science, the neuroplastic changes are considered both from a structural and functional level of adaptation; additionally, the two of them are interrelated as functional reorganization implies structural reorganization [11, 12]. On the one hand, thanks to several neuroimaging studies, music training is well known to be able to provoke anatomical as well as structural plastic changes even in the adult human brain [13]. A plethora of structural differences, manifested as increased gray matter volume, have been seen throughout literature in somatosensory areas, premotor cortex, inferior temporal and frontal regions, and in cerebellum in the brains of musicians compared to nonmusicians; results from longitudinal studies, in particular, showed a link between the duration of musical training and the degree of structural change in white matter pathways, such as the corpus callosum, highlighting the importance of reiterating the training over the years to see the long-term effects clearly [14–17]. Moreover, diffusion tensor imaging studies show greater structural connectivity after music training in other areas, such as in structures connecting visual and auditory brain areas located in the left inferior fronto-occipital fasciculus and connecting auditory and motor regions (e.g., arcuate fasciculus) as well as multimodal integration regions [18, 19]. In line with this, anatomical brain differences have been also found in auditory and motor cortices in relation to music training [13]. These findings reveal music-trained people to have specific brain areas that appear different compared to the starting age of music training. For example, a study with magnetic resonance imaging identified the left superior temporal gyrus, bilateral putamen (extending also to hippocampus and amygdala), and right thalamus as the regions linked with music training, in terms of cumulative hours of music lessons [20].

On the other hand, subtle functional changes, intended as deep modifications of synaptic strength in spread cortical networks, can be detected at a macrostructural and microstructural level after having music training or musical experience [12]. This brain adaptation through neurogenesis leads to changes also in behavioral performance, as demonstrated by studies showing correlations between brain changes and enhanced skills, i.e., auditory discrimination, motor sequencing, and speech skills [21, 22]. In sum, structural and functional changes due to musical experience take place at various stages of the auditory pathway, from the brainstem to primary and surrounding auditory cortices, to areas involved in higher-order auditory cognition [23]. This is confirmed by evidence that older people who have received long-term music training early in life have faster neural performance and timing on cognitive tasks, as well as increased auditory attention and executive functions [24, 25]. Similarly, an active music-based intervention is able to involve more analogous components to music training and learning, as it consists of the repeated practice of movements accompanied by auditory feedback and extensive cognitive processing. This explains the inclination of an active musical intervention to act as a multisensory stimulus, which makes it a useful tool for rehabilitation and prevention [11].

Findings on listening to music effects on the brain have been also useful to implement its use in healthcare environments. In particular, neurochemical research has revealed neurotransmitters' role on the affective components of listening to enjoyable music, namely their release of dopamine in the mesolimbic striatal system, as well as sensory regions for auditory reception together with peaks in autonomic nervous system activity [26, 27]. This may probably help to explain why music is so used for mood regulation and to achieve short-term enhancement of certain abilities in clinical settings. Indeed, even just exposure to listening to favorite music or songs with certain structural characteristics (e.g., fast pace and major mode) induces a state of greater activation capable of temporarily expand emotional resources and improving cognitive and motor performance (such as psychomotor speed, verbal fluency, and episodic memory) also in older people [28].

However, music listening can also lead to longer-term beneficial effects. Importantly, the neuroplastic modifications are not limited to the regular motor practice with an instrument, as merely listening to music during days, or even hours and minutes, can result in alterations of the brain functioning. This is due to the fact that listening to music under certain conditions (e.g., during aware and nonpassive listening where music is not used as a mere background) is characterized by the activation of dorsomedial prefrontal and occipital areas, thus eliciting an attentive internal state that allows for the initial reactions to sounds to become available for conscious evaluation [29]. Furthermore, music listening involves the drive to move and the memory process provoking network changes in the temporo-frontal brain areas and the hippocampus. As a result, when we listen, an automatic processing of repeated melodic and rhythmic patterns occurs together with the subsequent recognition [30].

Besides music, other forms of rehabilitative interventions able to induce neuroplastic changes have been recently explored. Similarly to musical interventions, noninvasive brain stimulation techniques have demonstrated the ability to modulate the neuronal excitability with a view to influencing plasticity mechanisms inherent in the central nervous system and temporarily improving a range of functions [31]. There are several forms of noninvasive brain stimulation, although the most widely adopted in the clinical setting is transcranial electrical stimulation (tEs). This technique consists of delivering a small (1–2 mA) current via two electrodes placed on the scalp. According to the stimulation parameters, tEs affects neural excitability and provokes plastic effects mediated by NMDA receptors [32]. These currents, cathodic (−) or anodic (+), generate an electric field able to modulate spontaneous neural activity by interfering with the membrane potential of the underlying neuronal structures and thus inducing hyperpolarization (inhibiting effect) or depolarization (facilitating effect), respectively [33]. Again, as for music-based interventions, it is important to underline that the brain changes produced become more stable and lasting (long-term effects) when the stimulation is repeated several times, likewise according to the principles of neuroplasticity [34, 35]. The most recent studies make a hybrid use of music and brain stimulation techniques to cope with cognitive decline. The results show the combination of tEs and music-based interventions give a greater boost to neuroplasticity than each of them can give individually and thus represent a functional, complementary solution to other types of therapy [36, 37].

2. Music as a nonpharmacological treatment in pathological aging: from the most well-known interventions up to novel approaches

As known, music has been extensively tested as a nonpharmacological intervention due to its effectiveness, its being inexpensive, and its possibility to be widely and easily applicable to clinical settings for the rehabilitation of a variety of age-related pathologies. Thanks to the awareness of the effects of music on neuroplasticity, a number of active and passive innovative music-based interventions, such as those of Neurologic Music Therapy (NMT) [38] and similar methodologies, also combined with new technologies, have risen in the last decades in order to promote brain reorganization after trauma and vascular problem or handle with cognitive decline during neurodegeneration. So far, its most significant application as a rehabilitation tool has been with post-stroke and dementia patients. This is because the urgency dictated by the compelling diffusion of these pathologies inevitably has led to the implementation and search for strategies to limit the discomfort of patients in their daily lives. In fact, stroke and dementia are two of the most occurring diseases during old age as well as the leading causes of neurological disability and death worldwide [39]. Specifically, every year 14 million people suffer a stroke, a number expected to increase by 34% up to 2035 [40, 41]. As regards dementia, and especially for Alzheimer's disease (AD), the number of people living with dementia was estimated to stand at 55 million in 2019 and is expected to rise up to 139 million in 2050 [42].

Findings from studies investigating non-degenerative disease related to brain traumas or vascular problems indicate music to be an effective means mostly for motor and language rehabilitation [28]. As mentioned, behavioral outcomes and brain functioning are related to each other; this means that altered behavior is a reflection of altered brain circuits, necessitating neurological renormalization or strengthening of substitute, relatively unharmed networks. The neuroplasticity capacity of the brain, able to provoke reorganization at both cortical and subcortical level, thus serves as the foundation for musical approaches to neurorehabilitation. Indeed, through the use of numerous pertinent neural circuits that are largely still guarded in the individual, music, which is a multimodal entity that engages perception, cognition, and motor control in the brain, serves as an effective medium for rehabilitating impaired neurologic functions [43].

In the specific case of motor rehabilitation after stroke, the aim is to enhance motor functions and induce and modulate plasticity through two main approaches: task-specific training (i.e., therapeutic interventions requiring the patient actively engage in motor skill re-learning guided by a therapist) and enriched environment; this latter consists of creating an engaging environment that promotes multimodal sensory processing as a result of physical, cognitive, and social activities [44]. Music-based active interventions for motor rehabilitation, which basically consists of playing musical instruments, encompass both approaches. Among them, one of the most investigated in recent times is the Music-Supported Therapy (MST) [45]. MST requires an electronic keyboard and an electronic drum set to train fine (keyboard) and gross (drums) movements, respectively. It is based on the principles of massive repetition, auditory-motor coupling and integration (i.e., reinforcement of motor effects due to immediate auditory feedback), shaping, tailoring the training to each individual's progress and emotion-motivation effects, which aids the rehabilitation process by engaging the reward-learning system. Several studies have proven its effectiveness in both acute and chronic stroke patients [46, 47]; see Grau-Sánchez et al. [48] for a review. These results, moreover, match with further experimental studies reporting brain changes in stroke patients after MST, therefore confirming and explaining the reasons behind the favorable outcomes of this technique from the neuroplasticity point of view. In particular, an increase in the excitability and a cortical motor map reorganization in the sensorimotor cortex was found [49] together with an intrahemispheric reorganization within the lesioned hemisphere after the training [50] indicating a re-establishment of functional connectivity between auditory and motor regions.

Another often compromised post-stroke area is that of language. Indeed, up to 40% of stroke patients experience post-stroke aphasia, a severe condition that affects speech production and/or understanding. It has a catastrophic effect on individuals, as it leads to lower quality of life more than any other stroke-related impairment due to patients' reduced participation and involvement in a range of life activities when in such condition, with a consequent predisposition to depression [51]. Among the most used music-based intervention designed for speech and language rehabilitation is the NMT technique named "Melodic Intonation Therapy" (MIT). In MIT, differences and commonalities between singing and speaking are used for a therapeutic scope: patients gradually shift from singing to speaking by intoning or singing common phrases while tapping their left hand rhythmically, and the musical prosody of the functional phrases or brief statements they sing or intone closely resemble the verbal utterance's typical speech inflection patterns [38]. The effectiveness of MIT has been proven by several RCTs, e.g., [52, 53]. It certainly depends, first of all, on the constructive use of the functions shared between speaking and singing during the intervention, i.e., the acoustical perception and production features as well as the ability of both systems to embed communicative functions in the auditory modality [54]. Secondly, MIT power comes from its ability to induce neuroplasticity in the damaged left hemisphere, together with greater activation in the right fronto-temporal regions and an increased functional connectivity between motor and right homologous language regions [55–57]. Hence, according to these findings, MIT is able to recruit undamaged homologous networks, compensating for affected speech function and help functional recovery of the compromised area. As already proposed by other authors [28, 58], both MST and MIT are optimal rehabilitation strategies able to promote behavioral benefits in elderly patients that still need to be grounded within a neurobiological understanding, as they are based on central nervous adaptations related to brain plasticity, therefore to neurobiological mechanisms underlying these beneficial effects.

In addition to MIT, a novel approach for language rehabilitation based on a passive music-based intervention for this type of patients, consisting in listening to vocal music, has been explored by more recent research [59, 60]. Previous pivotal studies on listening to music in post-stroke patients had already reported an enhancement of a range of cognitive abilities through the increase of gray matter volume in frontolimbic regions [61, 62]. In the case of vocal music listening, an interesting hypothesis is that it induces neuroplasticity effects on the language network in those brain areas linked to connected speech after stroke, such as the left frontal regions and their underlying white matter tracts [63]. Initial findings from the first studies on this topic are confirming this hypothesis: by one side, vocal music listening compared to audiobook listening would enhance the structural connectivity frontal aslant tract, i.e., an important tract for speech production [59]. On the other side, it would improve verbal memory by inducing changes in the longitudinal functional connectivity in the language network [60]. These discoveries corroborate the theory that language network engagement can be modulated by music and add new information on the empowering effect provoked by listening to music with sung lyrics. Thus, according to these findings, vocal music would be able to connect linguistic and musical information into a unified representation, through involvement by vocal music of bilateral frontotemporal areas in a more extensive way than speech alone. In general, given the encouraging results coming from research so far, it would be highly desirable to incorporate these techniques into post-stroke rehabilitation programs. Starting from the broad plastic potential for the brain language areas up to the involvement of motivation and reward circuits useful for enhancing motor functions, they constitute an excellent tool for functional, cognitive, and behavioral recovery of patients after stroke.

Considering tactics to promote brain plasticity in clinical settings could make a significant contribution to intervention strategies for healing and enhancement of functions; this could also provide people with hope for personal empowerment, as modern neuroscience largely shows the possibility for enhancing brain plasticity [64]. However, in the case of neurodegenerative pathologies like AD, halting cognitive decline is not feasible. Although, it is possible in any case to implement nonpharmacologic strategies to alleviate the symptoms and improve the life quality of demented patients, through stimulating leisure activities able to aid their cognitive and emotional capacity. Indeed, so far music-based interventions with AD patients have been implemented to deal with a variety of related disorders: progressive cognitive decline, memory impairment, visuospatial ability, executive function, language and speech production as well as behavioral and psychological symptoms, i.e., depression, anxiety, apathy, agitation, emotional control deficits, and sleep disorders which often lead to have problems living independently [65, 66]. One of the most effective and implemented music-based interventions with AD patients consists in a passive intervention of listening to familiar, popular, or autobiographical music in order to recall music-evoked emotions and music-evoked autobiographical memories [67–69] and to help patients to restore their sense of identity. This is because musical memory, intended as a special type of semantic memory, appears to be relatively preserved in

AD patients, differently from verbal and episodic memory. By consequence, patients experiment with a sense of familiarity for a melodic progression regardless of timbre, starting pitch and memory of a past event where the melody was heard, being able to recognize a particular musical piece in any key and at any tempo [70, 71]. Hence, during a music therapy session, it is possible to play the music they prefer both through technological means and/or by singing or playing musical instruments, since the mode difference will not affect the melody retrieval in memory.

At a neuroplastic level, as mentioned, listening to music is an intervention type with a great positive effect on cognitive function as it integrates perception of sounds, rhythms, and lyrics and the response to the sound requiring attention to an environment, which implies the simultaneous activation of cortical brain areas [29, 30, 65]. Furthermore, two more studies carried out with AD patients showed specific brain changes after several times of listening to preferred or long-known music. In one of them, the authors found an activation of brain regions involved in autobiographical memory (e.g., bilateral network of prefrontal, emotional, motor, auditory, and subcortical regions like cerebellum, putamen, and limbic structures) providing a potential mechanism by which the repeated activation of such areas can preserve musical memory and lead to improvements in overall memory [72]. In the other one, increases in functional connectivity in corticocortical and corticocerebellar networks have been found after the presentation of preferred musical stimuli, suggesting the possibility of improvements in brain network synchronization [73].

Music therapy has been included in the last Alzheimer's Disease International report [42] within the section named "Current and future non-pharmacological intervention in dementia." In the document, a distinction between mild and advanced stages of the disease is operated according to the different relaxing or stimulating facets of music. This dual quality of music brings to music-based intervention an extraordinary support to neurodegenerative diseases. During the mild stage of dementia, when distress, depression, and anxiety are associated with the decrease of cognitive performances, passive interventions as receptive music therapy to achieve psycho-musical relaxation techniques are considered useful to reduce these disorders. On the contrary, in the advanced stage, when verbal communication declines and apathy becomes one of the biggest behavioral symptoms to contend with, music interventions such as singing workshops and choirs are considered very pertinent to fight against apathy and to stimulate verbal communication. Thus, at all stages of the pathology, receptive, or active musical interventions have complementary impacts. The course of symptoms is obviously a consequence of the progressive neurodegeneration. Along the degenerative process, BDNF levels change with an increase in the early stages and then a decrease in the late stages, reflecting a starting compensatory neuronal repair mechanism followed by an increased neuronal loss and the consequent severity of dementia [74]. Previous studies carried out in BDNF on mice suggest that music exposure induces a relaxing and anxiolytic effect by increasing BDNF levels in the hippocampus [75]. It can therefore be deduced that music exposure would be able to increase the BDNF concentration and the activation of BDNF downstream signaling also in humans, but at the moment it is a mere speculation awaiting confirmation and empirical evidence. In that case, it would be possible to provide a molecular explanation for the role played by music in dementia and better understand the molecular mechanisms behind music effects on brain plasticity and AD, as well as giving more solid ground to the design of treatments [76].

Thus far, repeated music-based interventions have been observed to have long-term effects in both stroke (3 months) and dementia (2 months) [61, 77, 78]. This is because a stimulation repetition, including music stimulation, allows for persisting change in the strength of the synapse. This change takes place due to brief high-frequency stimulations enhancing the synaptic activity between two neurons. This causes a mechanism of long-term potentiation (LTP), which is mediated by NMDA glutamate receptors and leads to the strengthening of neuronal circuits at synaptic level. Specularly, the opposite effect has been defined as long-term depression (LTD), also involving NMDA receptors and occurring during longtime low rate stimulation. Contrary to LTP, LTD leads to decreased synaptic activity and weakening of synaptic connections [79, 80]. Both of these processes are neural mechanisms that underlie learning and memory and mostly occur in the hippocampus, which has been discovered to have indirect functional connections with the central auditory pathway, the fronto-medial cortex and, of course, with the remaining components of the limbic system [81]. These networks are involved in the formation of auditory memory and, in turn, auditory cues are involved in the formation of spatial memories [43, 82]. In sum, repeated sound stimulation and music are able to induce the LTP process, leading to an increase of BDNF levels and thus enhancing learning and memory abilities, which will be crucial for a comprehensive recovery of functional, cognitive, and behavioral aspects. Such awareness should therefore lead to a novel model of music therapy based on neuroplasticity, as claimed by a previous theoretical work by Stegemoller explaining how music therapy works on the brain through dopamine increase, neural synchrony, and a clear signal in contrast to noise [83]. In this regard, it is necessary to advance the production of empirical evidence and experiment new approaches capable of reinforcing and making the efficacy of music in clinical contexts even more evident.

2.1 Music and brain stimulation: when unity is strength

The principle of neuroplasticity through repetition is obviously applicable to other types of stimulation besides music. Periodical noninvasive brain stimulation is able to induce excitability changes of the cortex similar to the long-lasting LTP and LTD mechanism. On a behavioral level, these neuroplastic changes can be observed in a temporary improvement of some skills' performance [84–86]. This especially applies to transcranial direct current stimulation (tDCS), one of the noninvasive brain stimulation approaches that increasingly gather attention as a means for increasing or decreasing cortical excitability, depending on the delivery of anodal or cathodal stimulation to the cerebral cortex. This method has advantages over other transcranial stimulation techniques, such as its ease of application, the lower cost, and more prolonged modulating effect on the cerebral cortex; studies on its efficacy in post-stroke patients are emerging [87], as well as initial evidence on the positive effects on cognitive and psychiatric of patients with dementia [88, 89]. Some pioneering studies had shown a positive relationship between tDCS and auditory, motor, and visual processing, thanks to induced changes in the auditory cortex [90, 91]. Even newer are the applications of brain stimulation in hybrid rehabilitation approaches, especially in combination with music. Two recent studies with elderly participants combining tDCS and passive music-based intervention hypothesized that listening to autobiographically salient music is able to amplify the effects of tDCS on cognitive skills and corresponding brain functions [36, 37]. Specifically, in their study, Chow et al. [36] found personalized music to have the power to amplify the effects of tDCS for working memory (WM). Indeed, the combination may modulate neural processing of recognition memory when memory demands are high. Similarly, the study by Bidelman et al. [37] showed that tDCS paired with music listening can be a viable intervention to boost cognitive and WM performance, and in turn, receptive communication skills that decline during the lifespan. Listening to music and particularly to songs that evoke autobiographical memories would be then able to enhance responsivity to the effects of tDCS for older adults. This larger effect of the combination music+tDCS than music or tDCS alone supports previous findings in the literature demonstrating an advantage of combining tDCS with other cognitive tasks to maximize neuroplastic effects [92]. Although participants in these two studies were healthy elderly people, these findings are promising as they may have potential utility for clinical older adult populations who demonstrate a need for novel cognitive rehabilitation strategies, especially for individuals with AD and other dementias.

Further investigations also tried to combine tDCS with a range of music-based interventions, including active interventions. Two studies investigated the neuroplastic changes induced by tDCS by combining repeated sessions of anodal stimulation of the left temporal cortex with sound therapy (tailor-made notched music training) [93] or hearing aids [94], but neither study found any additional effect of tDCS to the audiological treatment [95]. Many other studies investigated the use of tDCS on the left temporoparietal cortex to treat the chronic subjective tinnitus [94, 96, 97] but were also negative. Other studies were designed to target the dorsolateral prefrontal cortex, which is involved in the tinnitus pathophysiology [98, 99] as well as major depression, which is a frequent comorbid disorder in tinnitus [100]. In a study by Moossavi et al. [101], they combined tDCS and tailor-made notched music training [102], a technique based on the hemostasis mechanism which induces the asynchrony in neural activities by lateral inhibition of neurons coding the notch area of the tinnitus frequency [103], which reduces the auditory cortex hyperactivities [102]. In their research, they found that tDCS, in combination with the tailor-made notched music training, was effective to reduce the loudness, awareness, and annoyance caused by tinnitus in the short term for up to more than a month after the end of the treatment. Additionally, this combined method revealed improvement of cognitive abilities such as auditory divided attention, auditory selective attention, and WM [101]. Music therapy and electric stimulation have been also used in the rehabilitation of aphasia. In their paper, Aravantinou-Fatorou et al. [104] divided their aphasic patients into three groups: group A, who did not perform music therapy and had no tDCS; group B, with only music therapy; and group C, which had a combined treatment with daily music therapy and tDCS. They found that when music therapy and tDCS were added to the rehabilitation program, the group C (32.6%) recovered to a greater extent than those patients in groups B (24.4%) and A (6.1%) [104]. A similar result has been achieved by Vines et al. [105] by combining MIT with a tDCS applied to the posterior inferior frontal gyrus of the right hemisphere in patients with Broca's aphasia. Results of their study show a greater improvement of language fluency in patients with a combined MIT + tDCS than those who had MIT + sham tDCS.

Overall, despite the little empirical evidence still available, it can be deduced that the synergy between music-based interventions (both active and passive) and brain stimulation represents an added value to more traditional therapeutic approaches. The capacity of both to promote neuroplasticity, together with the enriched environment and the rewarding stimuli provided by music therapy in clinical setting, able of creating an engaging environment and promoting multimodal sensory processing, can really constitute a resource and a model of therapy, based on neurobiological foundations, for the well-being of the elderly person.

2.2 Music meets technology: a glimpse into the future of rehabilitation

The inclusion of new technologies in active and passive music therapy sessions is actually already well known. With the evolution of technology and the need to find alternative therapeutic approaches to different disorders, the combination of traditional and innovative therapeutic techniques has become an important research approach. Starting with the implementation of music therapy interventions by the means of electronic devices [106], music technology has developed further in recent years providing both post-stroke and demented patients a variety of tools for rehabilitation, intersecting different research areas such as music psychology, neuroscience, music therapy, music information retrieval, music technology, medical technology, and robotics [107]. Such tools give the chance, for example, to combine sensors with MIDI converters to engage and stimulate consistent motor performance within improvisation as part of motor rehabilitation after stroke. Often, the movement location is translated to pitch height, offering an extra awareness of reach distance. In some other cases, percussion feedback sounds on bespoke instruments are used, allowing stroke patients to rehabilitate by drumming along to their own preferred music [108]. Recently, for AD patients, the effectiveness of interactive music exergames has been also explored to improve or maintain their physical condition while recovering past memories and an interest in social interaction [109].

The most significant innovation, probably, comes from another type of technological intervention, increasingly used in clinical settings and investigated by research in recent times, i.e., that based on virtual reality (VR), also indicated as an effective tool for older adults and able to induce neuroplasticity [110]. The progress and development of new devices to produce VR and augmented reality (AR) allow therapeutic interventions for a wide range of disorders [111]. Moreover, the customization and the possibility of using this type of technology make it possible to obtain low-cost and widely used therapeutic hardware and software. Some of the research areas in which the combination of music therapy and VR has produced greater results concern the management of anxiety states and in the palliative care of pain [112–114]. The results from these studies show how the combination of music therapy (in particular, the use of musical pieces linked to the preferences of the individual subjects) and VR has proved to be a feasible, usable, and acceptable tool for the improvement of states of anxiety and pain, highlighting more in general an improvement in the mood of the subjects. Furthermore, a use of these hybrid techniques has approached the treatment of neurodegenerative disorders, with particular interest in the different forms of dementia. The results show how the use of VR and music therapy can be a functional and complementary solution to other nonpharmacological therapies [115, 116]. Similarly to this approach, one of our team's research interventions will involve the use of VR in combination with music therapy on patients with different levels of cognitive impairment. In detail, the subjects will take part in a virtual environment experiment with familiar auditory and visual stimuli. Subjects will also undergo various tests to measure cognitive reserve before and after the intervention [117]. The principal aim is to evaluate neuroplastic processes and their modulation through the combination of musical and technological strategies, with a view to cope with cognitive decline and for a functional life.

3. Not only rehabilitation: the importance of prevention with music for a good elderly life

As known, the early stages of life are pivotal to maximize brain development in order to promote lifelong neuronal enrichment and accumulate what is referred to as "cognitive reserve." Nevertheless, it is important to promote brain plasticity throughout the life span. In this regard, researchers are starting to focus on the opportunity to induce neuroplasticity in the critical period of aging and underline how crucial it is to design engaging environments for the elderly that include activities able to support lifelong brain plasticity, emotional well-being, social bonding, and autonomy in everyday life [58]. A number of studies already exist on healthy older adults, e.g., [36, 37], providing both strategies for rehabilitation and findings on the potential cognitive protection of music. However, it is necessary to start thinking about elderly age not only from a rehabilitation perspective but also from a preventive point of view. In fact, there is a gap in research exploring the potential implications of music's long-term influence on neuroplasticity and music as a preventive measure to protect against impairment [11].

A good starting point in order to follow this direction is the literature available so far indicating that both music listening and active musical making, done regularly and frequently, have positive effects on the overall life of sick and healthy elderly. Music listening can facilitate cognitive, emotional, and neural recovery after stroke and support cognitive functioning, mood, and quality of life (QOL) in demented patients [61, 65]. Active music making, like playing an instrument, singing, and dancing have been shown to enhance executive functions, mood, and QOL in aged adults [118–122]. As seen, on the one hand, listening to autobiographical music restores the elderly's sense of identity and helps him/her to access memory through the emotions evoked by music. On the other hand, musical activities help older adults to connect with other people, increasing their self-esteem and decreasing feelings of isolation and loneliness; they have an influence on levels of hormones such as cortisol and affect the autonomic nervous systems by decreasing stress-related activation [123]. If regularly practiced, all musical activities offer great opportunities to maintain better mood and QOL and compensate for the gradual cognitive and neural decline associated with normal aging, potentially having a neuroprotective effect for neurodegenerative diseases. To transmute these deductions into empirical evidence, long-term studies with many years of follow-up, which are currently still lacking, and more research are needed on the topic.

4. Conclusions

Aging is a delicate phase of life characterized by psycho-physical decline and the onset of a variety of diseases provoked by neurodegenerative and vascular problems. According to research carried out mostly on clinical populations, such as on post-stroke and dementia patients, both active and passive music-based interventions have great rehabilitative potential and can constitute an optimal nonpharmacological treatment to be combined with traditional therapies. Moreover, neuroplasticity is now a well-established topic when studying the effects of music on the brain. Repetition over time of music listening and making is known to be able to induce neuroplastic changes and thus to provoke enhancement of a range of abilities on the behavioral level. Likewise, electrical brain stimulation techniques, including tDCS which is one of the most used, are able to induce long-term neuroplastic changes if repeated over time. A combination of music and brain stimulation, as well as music and other technology-based training like VR, is highly desirable in clinical settings with a view to innovative and more stimulating therapeutic offer. Moreover, it is important to ground the therapy with music on the model of neuroplasticity and, therefore, on the knowledge of neurobiological functions to a more effective implementation in healthcare environments. The hope is that music, with its positive functional, cognitive, emotional, and social influences and its innumerable possibilities of application, will be used as a stable tool for the well-being of the older person, not only in illness but also as a preventive and protective measure against impairment.

Acknowledgements

ML: Main writing of manuscript. FFC: Contribution to Section 2.1. FC: Contribution to Section 2.2. EB: Conception and contribution to overall writing and revision of the work.

Funding: Center for Music in the Brain (MIB) is funded by the Danish National Research Foundation (Project Number: 117). This research was supported by EU funding within the MUR PNRR A novel public-private alliance to generate socioeconomic, biomedical and technological solutions for an inclusive Italian ageing society (project n. PE00000015, AGE-IT).

Author details

Mariangela Lippolis[1], Francesco Carlomagno[1,2], Fulvia Francesca Campo[1,2] and Elvira Brattico[1,2]*

1 Department of Education, Psychology, Communication, University of Bari Aldo Moro, Bari, Italy

2 Department of Clinical Medicine, Center for Music in the Brain (MIB), Aarhus University and The Royal Academy of Music Aarhus/Aalborg, Aarhus, Denmark

*Address all correspondence to: elvira.brattico@clin.au.dk

References

[1] World Health Organization. International Day of Older Persons. 2022. Retrieved from: https://www.who.int/news-room/fact-sheets/detail/ageing-and-health

[2] Gramaglia C, Gattoni E, Marangon D, Concina D, Grossini E, Rinaldi C, et al. Non-pharmacological approaches to depressed elderly with No or mild cognitive impairment in long-term care facilities. A Systematic Review of Literature. Frontiers in Public Health. 2021;**9**:685860

[3] Toricelli M, Pereira AAR, Souza Abrao G, Malerba HN, Maia J, Buck HS, et al. Mechanisms of neuroplasticity and brain degeneration: Strategies for protection during the aging process. Neural Regeneration Research. 2021;**16**(1):58-67

[4] Satoh M, Ogawa J-i, Tokita T, Nakaguchi N, Nakao K, Kida H, et al. The effects of physical exercise with music on cognitive function of elderly people: Mihama-Kiho project. PLoS One. 2014;**9**(4):e95230

[5] Ferreri L, Moussard A, Bigand E, Tillmann B. Music and the aging brain. In: Thaut MH, Hodges DA, editors. The Oxford Handbook of Music and the Brain. Oxford, UK: Oxford University Press; 2019. pp. 623-644

[6] Maes PJ, Buhmann J, Leman M. 3Mo: A model for music-based biofeedback. Frontiers in Neuroscience. 2016;**10**:548

[7] Murray PS, Holmes PV. An overview of brain-derived neurotrophic factor and implications for excitotoxic vulnerability in the hippocampus. International Journal of Peptide. 2011;**2011**:654085

[8] Xing Y, Xia Y, Kendrick K, Liu X, Wang M, Wu D, et al. Mozart, Mozart rhythm and retrograde Mozart effects: Evidences from behaviours and neurobiology bases. Scientific Reports. 2016;**6**(1):1-11

[9] Chikahisa S, Sei H, Morishima M, Sano A, Kitaoka K, Nakaya Y, et al. Exposure to music in the perinatal period enhances learning performance and alters BDNF/TrkB signaling in mice as adults. Behavioural Brain Research. 2006;**169**:312-319

[10] Brattico E, Bonetti L, Ferretti G, Vuust P, Matrone C. Putting cells in motion: Advantages of endogenous boosting of BDNF production. Cell. 2021;**10**(1):1-16

[11] Schneider CE, Hunter EG, Bardach SH. Potential cognitive benefits from playing music among cognitively intact older adults: A scoping review. Journal of Applied Gerontology. 2019;**38**(12):1763-1178

[12] Reybrouck M, Vuust P, Brattico E. Music and Brain Plasticity: How Sounds Trigger Neurogenerative Adaptations. London, UK: Neuroplasticity—Insights of Neural Reorganization; 2018

[13] Olszewska AM, Gaca M, Herman AM, Jednoróg K, Marchewka A. How musical training shapes the adult brain: Predispositions and neuroplasticity. Frontiers in Neuroscience. 2021;**15**(Mar):1-16

[14] Moreno S, Bidelman GM. Examining neural plasticity and cognitive benefit through the unique lens of musical training. Hearing Research. 2013;**308**:84-97. DOI: 10.1016/j. heares.2013.09.012

[15] Barrett KC, Ashley R, Strait DL, Kraus N. Art and science: How musical

training shapes the brain. Frontiers in Psychology. 2013;**4**:713

[16] Miendlarzewska EA, Trost WJ. How musical training affects cognitive development: Rhythm, reward and other modulating variables. Frontiers in Neuroscience. 2014;7(8 JAN):1-18

[17] Criscuolo A, Pando-Naude V, Bonetti L, Vuust P, Brattico E. An ALE meta-analytic review of musical expertise. Scientific Reports. 2022;**12**:1-17

[18] Møller C, Garza-Villarreal EA, Hansen NC, Højlund A, Bærentsen KB, Chakravarty MM, et al. Audiovisual structural connectivity in musicians and non-musicians: A cortical thickness and diffusion tensor imaging study. Scientific Reports. 2021;**11**:1-14

[19] Schlaug G. Musicians and music making as a model for the study of brain plasticity. Progress in Brain Research. 2015;**217**:37-55

[20] Vaquero L, Hartmann K, Ripollés P, Rojo N, Sierpowska J, François C, et al. Structural neuroplasticity in expert pianists depends on the age of musical training onset. NeuroImage. 2016;**126**:106-119

[21] Hyde KL, Lerch J, Norton A, Forgeard M, Winner E, Evans AC, et al. Musical training shapes structural brain development. Journal of Neuroscience. 2009;**29**(10):3019-3025

[22] Bidelman GM, Villafuerte JW, Moreno S, Alain C. Age-related changes in the subcortical–cortical encoding and categorical perception of speech. Neurobiology of Aging. 2014;**35**(11):2526-2540

[23] Herholz SC, Zatorre RJ. Musical training as a framework for brain plasticity: Behavior, function, and structure. Neuron. 2012;**76**(3):486-502

[24] Bidelman GM, Alain C. Musical training orchestrates coordinated neuroplasticity in auditory brainstem and cortex to counteract age-related declines in categorical vowel perception. Journal of Neuroscience. 2015;**35**(3):1240-1249

[25] Sihvonen AJ, Särkämö T, Leo V, Tervaniemi M, Altenmüller E, Soinila S. Music-based interventions in neurological rehabilitation. The Lancet Neurology. 2017;**16**(8):648-660

[26] Zatorre RJ, Salimpoor VN. From perception to pleasure: Music and its neural substrates. Proceedings of the National Academy of Sciences of the USA. 2013;**110**:10430-10437

[27] Belfi A, Loui P. Musical anhedonia and rewards of music listening: Current advances and a proposed model. Annals of the New York Academy of Sciences. 2020;**1464**:99-114

[28] Särkämö T. Cognitive, emotional, and neural benefits of musical leisure activities in aging and neurological rehabilitation: A critical review. Annals of Physical and Rehabilitation Medicine. 2018;**61**(6):414-418

[29] Reybrouck M, Brattico E. Neuroplasticity beyond sounds: Neural adaptations following long-term musical aesthetic experiences. Brain Sciences. 2015;**5**(1):69-91

[30] Bonetti, L. Brattico, E. Carlomagno, F. Cabral, J. Stevner, A. Deco, G. Whybrow, P.C. Pearce, M. Pantazis, D. Vuust, P. et al. Spatiotemporal brain dynamics during recognition of the music of Johann Sebastian Bach. bioRxiv 2020;**165191**:1-44

[31] Filippetti M et al. Tecniche di stimolazione cerebrale non invasiva: la stimolazione elettrica transcranica. Revisione Narrativa Della Letteratura.

Giornale italiano di Medicina Riabilitativa. 2021;**36**(3):23-29

[32] Nitsche MA, Liebetanz D, Lang N, Antal A, Tergau F, Paulus W. Safety criteria for transcranial direct current stimulation (tDCS) in humans. Clinical Neurophysiology. 2003;**114**(11):2220-2222. author reply 2222-3

[33] Nitsche MA, Paulus W. Excitability changes induced in the human motor cortex by weak transcranial direct current stimulation. The Journal of Physiology. 2000;**527**(Pt 3):633

[34] Bolognini N, Pascual-Leone A, Fregni F. Using non-invasive brain stimulation to augment motor training-induced plasticity. Journal of Neuroengineering and Rehabilitation. 2009;**6**(1):1-13

[35] Kleim JA, Jones TA. Principles of experience-dependent neural plasticity: Implications for rehabilitation after brain damage. Journal of Speech, Language, and Hearing Research. 2008;**51**:S225-S239

[36] Chow R, Gandon AN, Moussard A, Ryan JD. Effects of transcranial direct current stimulation combined with listening to preferred music on memory in older adults. Scientific Reports. 2021;**11**(1):1-13

[37] Bidelman GM, Chow R, Noly-gandon A, Ryan JD, Bell KL, Rizzi R, et al. Transcranial direct current stimulation combined with listening to preferred music alters cortical speech processing in older adults. Frontiers in Neuroscience. 2022;**16**(July):1-13

[38] Thaut MH, McIntosh GC. Neurologic music therapy in stroke rehabilitation. Current Physical Medicine and Rehabilitation Reports. 2014;**2**(2):106?113

[39] Avan A, Hachinski V. Stroke and dementia, leading causes of neurological disability and death, potential for prevention. Alzheimer's Dement. 2021;**17**:1072-1076

[40] Johnson CO, Nguyen M, Roth GA, Nichols E, Alam T, Abate D, et al. Global, regional, and national burden of stroke, 1990-2016: A systematic analysis for the global burden of disease study 2016. Lancet Neurology. 2019;**18**:439-458

[41] Stevens E, Emmett E, Wang Y, McKevitt C, Wolfe C. The Burden of Stroke in Europe. Brussels, BE: Stroke Alliance for Europe; 2017

[42] Gauthier S, Webster C, Servaes S, Morais JA, Rosa-Neto P. World Alzheimer Report 2022: Life after Diagnosis: Navigating Treatment, Care and Support. London, England: Alzheimer's Disease International; 2022

[43] Chatterjee D, Hegde S, Thaut M. Neural plasticity: The substratum of music-based interventions in NeuroRehabilitation. 2021;**48**:155-166

[44] Liebermann DG, Buchman AS, Franks IM. Enhancement of motor rehabilitation through the use of information technologies. Clinical Biomechanics. 2006;**21**(1):8-20

[45] Schneider S, Schönle P, Altenmüller E, Münte T. Using musical instruments to improve motor skill recovery following a stroke. Journal of Neurology. 2007;**254**(10):1339-1346

[46] Rodriguez-Fornells A, Rojo N, Amengual JL, Ripolles P, Altenmuller E, Munte TF. The involvement of audio-motor coupling in the music-supported therapy applied to stroke patients. Annals of the New York Academy of Sciences. 2012;**1252**:282-293

[47] Ripollés P, Rojo N, Amengual JL, Càmara E. Music supported therapy

promotes motor plasticity in individuals with chronic stroke. Brain Imaging and Behavior. 2016;**10**(4):1289-1307

[48] Grau-Sánchez J, Münte TF, Altenmüller E, Duarte E, Rodríguez-Fornells A. Potential benefits of music playing in stroke upper limb motor rehabilitation. Neuroscience and Biobehavioral Reviews. 2020;**112**(February):585-599

[49] Grau-Sánchez J, Amengual JL, Rojo N, de Las V, Heras M, Montero J, et al. Plasticity in the sensorimotor cortex induced by music-supported therapy in stroke patients: A TMS study. Frontiers in Human Neuroscience. 2013;7:494

[50] Ripollés P, Rojo N, Grau-Sánchez J, Amengual JLL, Càmara E, Marco-Pallarés J, et al. Music supported therapy promotes motor plasticity in individuals with chronic stroke. Brain Imaging and Behavior. 2016;**10**(4):1289-1307

[51] Lam JMC, Wodchis WP. The relationship of 60 disease diagnoses and 15 conditions to preference-based health-related quality of life in Ontario hospital-based long-term care residents. Medical Care. 2010;**48**:380-387

[52] Van Der Meulen I, Van De Sandt-Koenderman MWME, Heijenbrok MH, Visch-Brink E, Ribbers GM. Melodic intonation therapy in chronic aphasia: Evidence from a pilot randomized controlled trial. Frontiers in Human Neuroscience. 2016;**10**:1-9

[53] Van Der Meulen I, Van De Sandt-Koenderman WME, Heijenbrok-Kal MH, Visch-Brink EG, Ribbers GM. The efficacy and timing of melodic intonation therapy in subacute aphasia. Neurorehabilitation and Neural Repair. 2014;**28**(6):536-544

[54] Thaut M, Koshimori Y. Neurorehabilitation in aging through neurologic music therapy. In: Music and the Aging Brain. Cambridge, MA, USA: Academic Press; 2020. pp. 351-382

[55] Breier JI, Randle S, Maher LM, Papanicolaou AC. Changes in maps of language activity activation following melodic intonation therapy using magnetoencephalography: Two case studies. Journal of Clinical and Experimental Neuropsychology. 2010;**32**(3):309-314

[56] Schlaug G, Marchina S, Norton A. From singing to speaking: Why singing may lead to recovery of expressive language function in patients with Broca's aphasia. Music Perception. 2008;**25**(4):315-323

[57] Bitan T, Simic T, Saverino C, Jones C, Glazer J, Collela B, et al. Changes in resting-state connectivity following melody-based therapy in a patient with aphasia. Neural Plasticity. 2018;**2018**:1-13

[58] Altenmüller E, James CE. The impact of music interventions on motor rehabilitation following stroke in elderly. In: Music and the Aging Brain. Cambridge, MA, USA: Academic Press; 2020. pp. 407-432

[59] Sihvonen AJ, Ripollés P, Leo V, Saunavaara J, Parkkola R, Rodríguez-Fornells A, et al. Vocal music listening enhances poststroke language network reorganization. ENeuro. 2021;**8**(4):1-10

[60] Sihvonen AJ, Pitkäniemi A, Leo V, Soinila S, Särkämö T. Resting-state language network neuroplasticity in post-stroke music listening: A randomized controlled trial. European Journal of Neuroscience. 2021;**54**(11):7886-7898

[61] Särkämö T, Tervaniemi M, Laitinen S, Forsblom A, Soinila S, Mikkonen M, et al. Music listening enhances cognitive recovery and mood

after middle cerebral artery stroke. Brain. 2008;**131**:866-876

[62] Särkämö T, Ripollés P, Vepsäläinen H, Autti T, Silvennoinen HM, Salli E, et al. Structural changes induced by daily music listening in the recovering brain after middle cerebral artery stroke: A voxel-based morphometry study. Frontiers in Human Neuroscience. 2014;**8**:245

[63] Alyahya RSW, Halai AD, Conroy P, Lambon MA. A unified model of post-stroke language deficits including discourse production and their neural correlates. Brain. 2020;**143**:1541-1554

[64] Shaffer J. Neuroplasticity and clinical practice: Building brain power for health. Frontiers in Psychology. 2016;7(Jul):1-12

[65] Moreno-Morales C, Calero R, Moreno-Morales P, Pintado C. Music therapy in the treatment of dementia: A systematic review and meta-analysis. Frontiers in Medicine. 2020;7(May):1-11

[66] Matziorinis AM, Koelsch S. The promise of music therapy for Alzheimer's disease: A review. Annals of the New York Academy of Sciences. 2022;**1516**(1):11-17

[67] Belfi AM, Karlan B, Tranel D. Music evokes vivid autobiographical memories. Memory. 2016;**24**(7):979-989

[68] Janata P, Tomic ST, Rakowski SK. Characterisation of music-evoked autobiographical memories. Memory. 2007;**15**:845-860

[69] El Haj M, Antoine P, Nandrino JL, Gély-Nargeot M-C, Raffard S. Self-defining memories during exposure to music in Alzheimer's disease. International Psychogeriatrics. 2015;**27**:1719-1730

[70] Peretz I, Coltheart M. Modularity of music processing. Nature Neuroscience. 2003;**6**:688-691

[71] Groussard M, Chan TG, Coppalle R, Platel H. Preservation of musical memory throughout the progression of Alzheimer's disease? Toward a reconciliation of theoretical, clinical, and neuroimaging evidence. Journal of Alzheimer's Disease. 2019;**68**(3):857-883

[72] Thaut MH, Fischer CE, Leggieri MM, Vuong V, Churchill NW, Fornazzari LR, et al. Neural basis of long-term musical memory in cognitively impaired older persons. Alzheimer Disease & Associated Disorders. 2020;**34**(3):267-271

[73] King JB, Jones KG, Goldberg E, et al. Increased functional connectivity after listening to favored music in adults with Alzheimer dementia. The Journal of Prevention of Alzheimer's Disease. 2019;**6**:56-62

[74] Laske C, Stransky E, Leyhe T, Eschweiler GW, Wittorf A, et al. Stage-dependent BDNF serum concentrations in Alzheimer's disease. Journal of Neural Transmission. 2006;**113**:1217-1224

[75] Li WJ, Yu H, Yang JM, Gao J, Jiang H, et al. Anxiolytic effect of music exposure on BDNFMet/met transgenic mice. Brain Research. 2010;**1347**:71-79

[76] Matrone C, Brattico E. The power of music on Alzheimer's disease and the need to understand the underlying molecular mechanisms. Journal of Alzheimers Disease & Parkinsonism. 2015;**5**:196

[77] Särkämö T, Laitinen S, Numminen A, Kurki M, Johnson JK, Rantanen P. Pattern of emotional benefits induced by regular singing and music listening in dementia. Journal of the American Geriatrics Society. 2016;**64**(2):439-440

[78] Raglio A, Bellandi D, Baiardi P, et al. Effect of active music therapy and individualized listening to music on

dementia: A multicenter randomized controlled trial. Journal of the American Geriatrics Society. 2015;**63**(8):1534-1539

[79] Nicoll RA, Kauer JA, Malenka RC. The current excitement in longterm potentiation. Neuron. 1988;**1**(2):97-103

[80] Mulkey RM, Malenka RC. Mechanisms underlying induction of homosynaptic long-term depression in area CA1 of the hippocampus. Neuron. 1992;**9**(5):967-975

[81] Rocchi F, Oya H, Balezeau F, Billig AJ, Kocsis Z, Jenison RL, et al. Common fronto-temporal effective connectivity in humans and monkeys. Neuron. 2021;**109**(5):852-868

[82] Dietz B, Manahan-Vaughan D. Hippocampal long-term depression is facilitated by the acquisition and updating of memory of spatial auditory content and requires mGlu5 activation. Neuropharmacology. 2017;**115**:30-41

[83] Stegemoller EL. Exploring a neuroplasticity model of music therapy. Journal of Music Therapy. 2014;**51**(3):211-227

[84] Monte-Silva K, Kuo MF, Hessenthaler S, Fresnoza S, Liebetanz D, Paulus W, et al. Induction of late LTP-like plasticity in the human motor cortex by repeated non-invasive brain stimulation. Brain Stimulation. 2013;**6**(3):424-432

[85] Hsu W-Y, Zanto TP, Anguera JA, Lin Y-Y, Gazzaley A. Delayed enhancement of multitasking performance: Effects of anodal transcranial direct current stimulation on the prefrontal cortex. Cortex. 2015;**69**:175-185

[86] Kronberg G, Bridi M, Abel T, Bikson M, Parra LC. Direct current stimulation modulates LTP and LTD: Activity dependence and dendritic effects. Brain Stimulation. 2017;**10**(1):51-58

[87] Satow T, Kawase T, Kitamura A, Kajitani Y, Yamaguchi T, Tanabe N, et al. Combination of transcranial direct current stimulation and neuromuscular electrical stimulation improves gait ability in a patient in chronic stage of stroke. Case Reports in Neurology. 2016;**8**(1):39-46

[88] Inagawa T, Narita Z, Sugawara N, Maruo K, Stickley A, Yokoi Y, et al. A meta-analysis of the effect of multisession transcranial direct current stimulation on cognition in dementia and mild cognitive impairment. Clinical EEG and Neuroscience. 2019;**50**(4):273-282

[89] Ferrucci R, Mrakic-Sposta S, Gardini S, Ruggiero F, Vergari M, Mameli F, et al. Behavioral and neurophysiological effects of transcranial direct current stimulation (tDCS) in fronto-temporal dementia. Frontiers in Behavioral Neuroscience. 2018;**12**:235

[90] Nitsche MA, Cohen LG, Wassermann EM, Priori A, Lang N, Antal A, et al. Transcranial direct current stimulation: State of the art 2008. Brain Stimulation. 2008;**1**(3):206-223

[91] Impey D, Knott V. Effect of transcranial direct current stimulation (tDCS) on MMN-indexed auditory discrimination: A pilot study. Journal of Neural Transmission. 2015;**122**(8):1175-1185

[92] Assecondi S, Shapiro K. The benefits of combined brain stimulation and cognitive training: A pilot study. Journal of Vision. 2018;**18**:119-119

[93] Teismann H, Wollbrink A, Okamoto H, Schlaug G, Rudack C, Pantev C. Combining transcranial direct current stimulation and tailor-made

notched music training to decrease tinnitus-related distress–a pilot study. PLoS One. 2014;**9**(2):e89904

[94] Shekhawat GS, Searchfield GD, Stinear CM. Randomized trial of transcranial direct current stimulation and hearing aids for tinnitus management. Neurorehabilitation and Neural Repair. 2014;**28**(5):410-419

[95] Lefaucheur JP, Antal A, Ayache SS, Benninger DH, Brunelin J, Cogiamanian F, et al. Evidence-based guidelines on the therapeutic use of transcranial direct current stimulation (tDCS). Clinical Neurophysiology. 2017;**128**(1):56-92

[96] Forogh B, Mirshaki Z, Raissi GR, Shirazi A, Mansoori K, Ahadi T. Repeated sessions of transcranial direct current stimulation for treatment of chronic subjective tinnitus: A pilot randomized controlled trial. Neurological Sciences. 2016;**37**(2):253-259

[97] Hyvärinen P, Mäkitie A, Aarnisalo AA. Self-administered domiciliary tDCS treatment for tinnitus: A double-blind sham-controlled study. PLoS One. 2016;**11**(4):e0154286

[98] Vanneste S, De Ridder D. Bifrontal transcranial direct current stimulation modulates tinnitus intensity and tinnitus-distress-related brain activity. European Journal of Neuroscience. 2011;**34**(4):605-614

[99] Joos K, Vanneste S, De Ridder D. Disentangling depression and distress networks in the tinnitus brain. PLoS One. 2012;**7**(7):e40544

[100] Langguth B, Landgrebe M, Kleinjung T, Sand GP, Hajak G. Tinnitus and depression. The World Journal of Biological Psychiatry. 2011;**12**(7):489-500

[101] Moossavi A, Mehrkian S, Najafi S, Bakhshi E. The effectiveness of the combined transcranial direct current stimulation (tDCS) and tailor-made notched music training (TMNMT) on psychoacoustic, psychometric, and cognitive indices of tinnitus patients. American Journal of Otolaryngology. 2022;**43**(1):103274

[102] Pantev C, Okamoto H, Teismann H. Music-induced cortical plasticity and lateral inhibition in the human auditory cortex as foundations for tonal tinnitus treatment. Frontiers in Systems Neuroscience. 2012;**6**:50

[103] Pantev C, Rudack C, Stein A, Wunderlich R, Engell A, Lau P, et al. Study protocol: münster tinnitus randomized controlled clinical trial-2013 based on tailor-made notched music training (TMNMT). BMC Neurology. 2014;**14**(1):1-8

[104] Aravantinou-Fatorou A, Georgakopoulou VE, Spandidos DA, Papalexis P, Tarantinos K, Mathioudakis N, et al. Effects of music therapy accompanied by transcranial direct current stimulation on the recovery from aphasia following stroke: A single-center retrospective cohort study. World Academy of Sciences Journal. 2022;**4**(6):1-9

[105] Vines BW, Norton AC, Schlaug G. Non-invasive brain stimulation enhances the effects of melodic intonation therapy. Frontiers in Psychology. 2011;**2**:230

[106] Magee WL, Burland K. An exploratory study of the use of electronic music technologies in clinical music therapy. Nordic Journal of Music Therapy. 2008;**17**(2):124-141

[107] Kirk P, Grierson M, Bodak R, Ward N, Brander F, Kelly K, et al. Motivating stroke rehabilitation through music: A feasibility study using digital musical instruments in the home [Conference paper]. In: Proceedings of

the 2016 CHI Conference on Human Factors in Computing Systems. New York, NY, United States: Association for Computing Machinery, San Jose, CA; 2016. pp. 1781-1785

[108] Agres KR, Schaefer RS, Volk A, van Hooren S, Holzapfel A, Dalla Bella S, et al. Music, computing, and health: A roadmap for the current and future roles of music technology for health care and well-being. Music & Science. 2021;**4**:2059204321997709

[109] Unbehaun D, Taugerbeck S, Aal K, Vaziri DD, Lehmann J, Tolmie P, et al. Notes of memories: Fostering social interaction, activity and reminiscence through an interactive music exergame developed for people with dementia and their caregivers. Human–Computer Interaction. NY, United States: Association for Computing Machinery, New York. 2021;**36**(5-6):439-472

[110] Huang K. Exergaming executive functions: An immersive virtual reality-based cognitive training for adults aged 50 and older. Cyberpsychology, Behavior and Social Networking. 2020;**23**(3):143-149

[111] Parsons TD, Rizzo AA. Affective outcomes of virtual reality exposure therapy for anxiety and specific pho-bias: A meta-analysis. Journal of Behavior Therapy and Experimental Psychiatry. 2008;**39**(3):250-261

[112] Brungardt A, Wibben A, Tompkins AF, Shanbhag P, Coats H, LaGasse B, et al. Virtual reality-based music therapy in palliative care: A pilot implementation trial. Journal of Palliative Medicine. 2021;**24**(5):736-742

[113] Cabezas CA, Arcos AR, Carrillo-Medina JL, Arias-Almeida GI. Effects of virtual reality and music therapy on academic stress reduction using a Mobile application. In: Botto-Tobar M, Gómez S, Rosero O, Miranda R, Díaz Cadena A, Montes León S, Luna-Encalada W, editors. Trends in Artificial Intelligence and Computer Engineering. ICAETT 2021. Lecture Notes in Networks and Systems. Vol. 407. Cham: Springer; 2022

[114] Chirico A, Maiorano P, Indovina P, Milanese C, Giordano GG, Alivernini F, et al. Virtual reality and music therapy as distraction interventions to alleviate anxiety and improve mood states in breast cancer patients during chemotherapy. Journal of Cellular Physiology. 2020;**235**(6):5353-5362

[115] Raglio A, Bellelli G, Mazzola P, Bellandi D, Giovagnoli AR, Farina E, et al. Music, music therapy and dementia: A review of literature and the recommendations of the Italian psychogeriatric association. Maturitas. 2012;**72**(4):305-310

[116] Byrns A, Abdessalem HB, Cuesta M, Bruneau MA, Belleville S, Frasson C. Adaptive music Ther-apy for Alzheimer's disease using virtual reality. In: International Conference on Intelligent Tutoring Systems. Cham: Springer; 2020. pp. 214-219

[117] Carlomagno F, Brattico E. Relieve Social Isolation and its Consequent Neurological Damage in Pathological Aging through Electrical and Musical Stimulation in a Virtual and Augmented Reality Environment (VR+AR). [Unpublished manuscript]. Bari, BA, IT: University of Bari Aldo Moro; 2023

[118] Coulton S, Clift S, Skingley A, Rodriguez J. Effectiveness and cost-effectiveness of community singing on mental health-related quality of life of older people: Randomised controlled trial. British Journal of Psychiatry. 2015;**207**:250-255

[119] Johnson JK, Louhivuori J, Stewart AL, Tolvanen A, Ross L, Era P. Quality of life (QOL) of older adult community choral singers in Finland. International Psychogeriatrics. 2013;**25**:1055-1064

[120] Bugos JA, Perlstein WM, McCrae CS, Brophy TS, Bedenbaugh PH. Individualized piano instruction enhances executive functioning and working memory in older adults. Aging & Mental Health. 2007;**11**:464-471

[121] Pentikäinen E, Pitkäniemi A, Siponkoski S-T, Jansson M, Louhivuori J, Johnson JK, et al. Beneficial effects of choir singing on cognition and well-being of older adults: Evidence from a cross-sectional study. PLoS ONE. 2021;**16**(2):e0245666

[122] James CE, Altenmüller E, Kliegel M, et al. Train the brain with music (TBM): Brain plasticity and cognitive benefits induced by musical training in elderly people in Germany and Switzerland, a study protocol for an RCT comparing musical instrumental practice to sensitization to music. BMC Geriatr. 2020;**20**:418

[123] de Witte M, Spruit A, van Hooren S, Moonen X, Stams GJ. Effects of music interventions on stress-related outcomes: A systematic review and two meta-analyses. Health Psychology Review. 2020;**14**(2):294-324